A SYSTEMATIC APPROACH TO EVALUATION OF NURSING PROGRAMS

SECOND EDITION

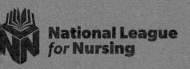
National League for Nursing

A SYSTEMATIC APPROACH TO EVALUATION OF NURSING PROGRAMS

SECOND EDITION

Edited by:

Marilyn H. Oermann, PhD, RN, FAAN, ANEF

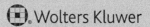

Wolters Kluwer

Philadelphia • Baltimore • New York • London
Buenos Aires • Hong Kong • Sydney • Tokyo

Vice President, Nursing Segment: Julie K. Stegman
Manager, Nursing Education and Practice Content: Jamie Blum
Senior Development Editor: Meredith L. Brittain
Marketing Manager: Sarah Schuessler
Editorial Assistant: Devika Kishore
Manager, Graphic Arts and Design: Steve Druding
Art Director: Jennifer Clements
Production Project Manager: Kirstin Johnson
Manufacturing Coordinator: Margie Orzech
Prepress Vendor: Aptara, Inc.

Oermann, M. H. (2023). *A systematic approach to evaluation of nursing programs* (2nd ed.). National League for Nursing.

9 8 7 6 5 4 3 2 1

Printed in the United States of America

Library of Congress Cataloging-in-Publication Data available upon request

ISBN: 978-1-9752-0619-2

shop.LWW.com   www.NLN.org

MPP0922

About the Editor

Marilyn H. Oermann, PhD, RN, FAAN, ANEF, is the Thelma M. Ingles Professor of Nursing and Director of Educational Research at Duke University School of Nursing, Durham, North Carolina. She is the editor-in-chief of *Nurse Educator*. Dr. Oermann is the author/co-author of 25 books, more than 210 articles in peer-reviewed journals, and many editorials, chapters, and other types of publications. Her current books are *Evaluation and Testing in Nursing Education; Writing for Publication in Nursing; Teaching in Nursing and Role of the Educator: The Complete Guide to Best Practice in Teaching, Evaluation, and Curriculum Development; and Clinical Teaching Strategies in Nursing.* Dr. Oermann is a fellow in the American Academy of Nursing and 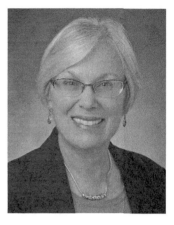 National League for Nursing (NLN) Academy of Nursing Education. She received the NLN Award for Excellence in Nursing Education Research and the President's Award, Sigma's Elizabeth Russell Belford Award for Excellence in Education, the American Association of Colleges of Nursing Scholarship of Teaching and Learning Excellence Award, and the Margaret Comerford Freda Award for Editorial Leadership in Nursing from the International Academy of Nursing Editors.

About the Contributors

Nicole Petsas Blodgett, PhD, RN, CHSE, is an assistant professor and director of the Center for Nursing Discovery at the Duke University School of Nursing in Durham, North Carolina. Dr. Blodgett has over 20 years of experience as a nurse educator. She was an International Nursing Association for Clinical Simulation and Learning Research Fellow (2018–2019), which led to a program of research related to the measurement of simulation faculty workload. She has served as a manuscript reviewer for *Clinical Simulation in Nursing* and the *Western Journal of Nursing Research* and has numerous peer-reviewed publications and presentations related to simulation design, operations, evaluation, and outcomes. Dr. Blodgett is a member of Sigma, the Society for Simulation in Healthcare, and the International Nursing Association for Clinical Simulation and Learning (INACSL) and serves on the INACSL Nominations and Elections Committee.

Lisa D. Brodersen, EdD, PhD, RN, CNE, is a professor and Coordinator of Institutional Research and Effectiveness at Allen College-UnityPoint Health, Waterloo, Iowa. Dr. Brodersen joined the faculty at Allen College in 1999 after working primarily in cardiac surgical intensive care for 16 years. She currently teaches evidence-based practice and biostatistics in the graduate nursing program and assists faculty and students in both nursing and health sciences programs with research and scholarly projects. Her professional activities include serving as a manuscript reviewer for several nursing education journals and reviewing conference abstracts and grant applications for the Midwest Nursing Research Society and Sigma. Dr. Brodersen's research interests include nursing education issues such as test-related stress and anxiety and student participation in nursing education research.

Kathy Casey, PhD, RN, NPD-BC, is a professional development specialist at Denver Health, in Denver, Colorado. Kathy is the coordinator of the Graduate Nurse Residency Program, which focuses on supporting and retaining graduate nurses as they transition into professional nursing practice. She is an assistant professor at the University of Colorado, College of Nursing, teaches Professional Role Development in the RN-BSN online program, and is a preceptor for DNP students completing their capstone projects at Denver Health. Her research endeavors include the development and testing of the Casey-Fink Graduate Nurse Experience Survey, a reliable and valid instrument designed to measure graduate nurse role transition into clinical practice. In addition, she co-developed the Casey-Fink Readiness for Practice Survey, designed to measure readiness for practice, and the Casey-Fink Nurse Retention survey, designed to measure nurse retention.

John M. Clochesy, PhD, MA, RN, is professor and director of evaluation and strategic initiatives at the University of Miami School of Nursing and Health Studies. Inducted as a fellow in the American Academy of Nursing and the American College of Critical Care Medicine, he has more than 40 years of experience as a nurse educator and researcher. He has authored more than 90 articles, 17 book chapters, 5 books, and was the founding Editor of *AACN Clinical Issues* (now *AACN Advanced Critical Care*).

Karen H. Frith, PhD, RN, NEA-BC, CNE, is professor of nursing and dean at the University of Alabama in Huntsville College of Nursing. She is board certified as a nurse executive, advanced, by the American Nurses Credentialing Center and is a certified nurse educator by the NLN. Dr. Frith has a notable scholarship record with over 60 peer-reviewed journal articles, 15 book chapters, and two books. She serves on the editoral board for *Nursing Education Perspectives*.

Kim Leighton, PhD, RN, CHSE, CHSOS, FSSH, FAAN, ANEF, is executive director of the Itqan Clinical Simulation and Innovation Center of Hamad Medical Corporation in Doha, Qatar. She currently serves on the board of directors for the Society for Simulation in Healthcare and is past president of the International Nursing Association on Clinical Simulation and Learning, where she spearheaded the development of the first Standards of Best Practice™ Simulation. Her research interests include evaluation of learning in clinical environments, with a focus on developing evaluation instruments for simulation-based learning. She is co-editor of the award winning book *Simulation Champions: Courage, Caring, and Connections*.

Lynne Porter Lewallen, PhD, RN, CNE, ANEF, is professor and associate dean for Academic Affairs in the School of Nursing at the University of North Carolina at Greensboro, Greensboro, North Carolina. She has experience with accreditation teams and review boards, and speaks and consults about program evaluation and accreditation. Her research interests include clinical evaluation and determination of competence in nursing education. Dr. Lewallen is a fellow in the Academy of Nursing Education, is a certified nurse educator, and serves on the editorial board of *Nursing Education Perspectives*.

Joan Such Lockhart, PhD, RN, CNE, FAAN, ANEF, is a tenured professor and director of the MSN Nursing Education Program at Duquesne University School of Nursing, Pittsburgh, Pennsylvania. As the former associate dean for academic affairs, she co-chaired the university's Academic Learning Outcomes Assessment Committee, led the school's program evaluation processes, and was instrumental in its successful accreditation and NLN Center of Excellence recognitions. Her teaching, scholarship, and service mirror her expertise in oncology, nursing professional development, and academic education, with a focus on caring for culturally diverse and vulnerable populations and developing a nursing workforce prepared to care for increasing numbers of cancer survivors. Dr. Lockhart is a fellow in the American Academy of Nursing and NLN Academy of Nursing Education, serves as the deputy editor for *The Journal of Continuing Education in Nursing* and Associate Editor for *ORL-Head and Neck Nursing*, and is on the editorial board of *Nurse Educator*. She recently authored *Nursing Professional Development for Clinical Educators* for the Oncology Nursing Society.

Jacquelyn McMillian-Bohler, PhD, CNM, CNE, is an assistant professor and the director of the Institute for Educational Excellence at Duke University School of Nursing. As a nurse educator with more than 20 years of experience at the master's and prelicensure levels, Dr. McMillian-Bohler is passionate about teaching and helping others achieve a masterful teacher practice. Her scholarship stems from her master teacher model and includes topics related to faculty development, teaching and learning strategies, and supporting an inclusive learning environment.

Melinda G. Oberleitner, DNS, RN, FAAN, is dean, College of Nursing and Health Sciences, and a professor in the LHC Group Myers School of Nursing at the University of Louisiana at Lafayette, Lafayette, Louisiana. She holds the LHC Group Endowed Deanship and the SLEMCO/BORSF Endowed Professorship in Nursing. Dr. Oberleitner has extensive experience in nursing education and academic program administration and has taught at the undergraduate and graduate levels for almost 40 years. Her teaching, scholarly publications, presentations, and funded grants have focused on nursing leadership and management, oncology nursing, and nursing education.

Teresa Shellenbarger, PhD, RN, CNE, CNEcl, ANEF, is the executive director of the National League for Nursing Commission for Nursing Education Accreditation (CNEA) in Washington, DC. She is a distinguished university professor emerita and previously served as the doctoral program coordinator at Indiana University of Pennsylvania, Indiana, Pennsylvania. During her 30 years as a nurse educator, she taught across various programs and levels of nursing education and has established a reputation as an expert educator and respected leader advocating for quality and excellence in nursing education. She is an NLN-certified academic nurse educator and clinical nurse educator and was inducted as an inaugural fellow in the NLN Academy of Nursing Education.

Theresa M. "Terry" Valiga, EdD, RN, CNE, FAAN, ANEF, is a professor emerita at Duke University School of Nursing, Durham, North Carolina, where she served as the director of the school's Institute for Educational Excellence and chair of the Division of Systems and Analytics. Immediately prior to her appointment at Duke, she served as the chief program officer at the NLN. She has published extensively on a variety of leadership and education-related topics, co-authored seven books, served on governing boards of several national organizations, presented papers and workshops at national and international conferences, and served as a consultant to many schools of nursing throughout the United States and in other countries. Dr. Valiga has received prestigious national awards including Sigma Theta Tau's Elizabeth Russell Belford Founders Award for Excellence in Nursing Education and the NLN's Outstanding Leadership in Nursing Education Award. She is a fellow of the Academy of Nursing Education and the American Academy of Nursing.

Diana M. Vergara, MA, is the director of assessment in the Office of University Accreditation for the University of Miami, Miami, Florida. She oversees the institutional assessment of the university's 300+ academic programs and service units, as well as the university's general education requirements and quality enhancement plan. Ms. Vergara has extensive experience in preparing self-study reports and accreditation site visits for nursing programs and other disciplines in both public and private universities. As an administrator, she works closely with faculty and program leaders in interpreting accreditation standards and improving or implementing new processes for compliance with accreditation and regulatory standards.

Foreword

The fourth core value of the National League for Nursing (NLN) is excellence, which we define as "co-creating and implementing transformative strategies with daring ingenuity." This book, edited by Marilyn H. Oermann, is a fine example of the implementation of this value. The co-creating happens as the editor, in partnership with other authors, navigates the field of formative and summative evaluation for schools of nursing. This develops the potential guided implementation and documented outcomes of program decision-making at schools of nursing throughout the United States and the global community.

As a significant missing piece of the puzzle for successful accreditation, steps to deliver ongoing evaluation for nursing programs represent truly transformative strategies. The strategies offered in this book, itemized in detail by expert faculty, can be used to change the culture for nursing programs attempting to seek successful accreditation. For programs that have already achieved accreditation, the strategies presented here will offer options for ongoing systematic evaluation that are based on evidence. We promote evidence-based nursing practice but do not yet have evidence-based nursing education programs. Our students deserve a culture of nursing school programs built on evidence, one that is vital for the successful transformation of our health care system and the well-being of our patients.

Colleagues, you will find the daring ingenuity of excellence in each of these chapters. Along with the accreditation of nursing programs, the chapters explore program and curriculum evaluation, collecting quality evaluation data, the development of systematic program evaluation plans for schools of nursing, the assessment of online courses and programs, the evaluation of specific program types, evaluation and accreditation of simulation programs, and the evaluation of educational programs in practice settings. You will find much more in these pages in this new edition for the nursing community.

This textbook touches the foundation of quality nursing education and will be useful for faculty and graduate students across all types of nursing programs. So, I am pleased to bring you excellence, from this book's outstanding editor, Dr. Oermann, and the incredible authors, all dedicated to transforming nursing education and fulfilling the mission of the NLN: The NLN promotes excellence in nursing education to build a strong and diverse nursing workforce to advance the health of the nation and global community.

Beverly Malone, PhD, RN, FAAN
President and CEO
The National League for Nursing

Preface

Program evaluation is a systematic process of collecting data for making decisions about a nursing program and judging its value. With the need to offer high-quality nursing programs and continued growth of new programs and delivery methods, systematic and ongoing program evaluation is critical across all schools of nursing and levels of education. Program evaluation not only provides data for decision making within an organization but also for accreditation.

The focus of this book is on evaluation of nursing programs, not the evaluation of individual students and their learning. The book provides under one cover the concepts that nurse educators should understand to engage in program evaluation and accreditation and includes examples and practical strategies for "getting it done." This second edition includes new chapters on evaluation and accreditation of simulation programs (Chapter 10) and on evaluation of educational programs in clinical practice settings (Chapter 11). Chapters from the first edition that are included in this new edition have been updated with new content and examples. The book was written for nurse educators, administrators, and others involved in program evaluation in all types of nursing programs and for nursing students in graduate courses that include program evaluation. Nurse educators in clinical settings who are responsible for developing and evaluating educational programs also will find the book helpful.

Chapter 1 provides an overview of program evaluation and describes its purposes, including differences between internal and external and between formative and summative evaluation. Three commonly used program evaluation models—Context, Input, Process, Product (CIPP); logic; and Kirkpatrick's four-level—are explained. Because the evaluation needs to provide the "right" information to make decisions about the program and to answer faculty, administrator, and other stakeholder questions, the process should be systematic, well planned, and ongoing. Steps to follow for a successful program evaluation are outlined in Chapter 1.

Faculty in schools of nursing spend a great deal of time designing the curriculum, implementing it in ways that engage the learner, and evaluating what students have learned as a result of those experiences. Efforts to evaluate the entire curriculum, however, are often overlooked, not approached in a systematic way, and incomplete. Chapter 2 addresses the purposes of and ways to approach curriculum evaluation, relates this activity to the overall program evaluation, and clarifies the role of faculty in the curriculum development, evaluation, and revision processes.

Program evaluation results are dependent on well-thought-out, relevant evaluation questions. These questions are often based on information needed for accreditation and to answer questions about the extent to which students are achieving the program outcomes and developing competencies. Evaluation questions are not the same as survey questions: Evaluation questions are broader and may require administering one or more surveys. Chapter 3 provides guidelines for writing good evaluation and good survey questions, identifying appropriate indicators, and creating high quality surveys. Examples are provided of various types of survey questions (open ended, closed ended, multiple choice, nominal response, ordinal response, numeric rating, Likert, matrix, and ranking). This chapter provides the information you need to write your evaluation questions and prepare your surveys for program evaluation.

The evaluation plan specifies the types of data to collect for program evaluation. Faculty rely on systematically collected quality data to make good decisions about their nursing program. Chapter 4 provides an overview of data and data sources frequently used in program evaluation. Psychometric considerations of reliability and validity, internal and external factors that have an impact on data quality, types of data collection methods for program evaluation, considerations when using existing assessment tools, and strategies for capturing data from key stakeholders are described in the chapter.

Chapter 5 describes the purposes of accreditation, types of accreditation, and typical program elements represented in accreditation standards for nursing education. The chapter also provides an overview of the accreditation process and explains the relationships among program evaluation, continuous quality improvement, and the accreditation process.

Systematic program evaluation is critical for program improvement as well as adherence to regulatory and accreditation standards. Chapter 6 discusses the rationale for program evaluation and how to get started in creating a program evaluation plan or revising an existing plan. Areas to include in a plan are described, and examples of completed evaluation plans are included in Appendix A to illustrate strategies to evaluate selected criteria.

The process of accreditation is rigorous, and preparing for accreditation can be overwhelming. Chapter 7 offers specific guidelines and helpful tips in preparing for the accreditation process. The authors describe who should be involved, the timeframe, setting up processes for accreditation, collecting and organizing the data, writing the self-study, preparing for a site visit (on-site or virtual), organizing the document room (including developing a digital resource room), and potential challenges.

Assessment of online courses and programs is an integral part of a nursing program's systematic program evaluation plan. Regardless of the level of course or academic degree, guidelines and approaches have been developed that can promote effective evaluation. Chapter 8 addresses evaluating online courses, establishing benchmarks for program success, and assessing the quality of courses and programs using valid and reliable tools. In addition, the chapter discusses the issues related to nursing courses and programs offered in other states and impact on evaluation and accreditation.

Chapter 9 focuses on specific types of nursing programs: RN to BSN, accelerated second career, nurse practitioner, nurse anesthetist, and doctoral nursing programs. These programs have unique assessment needs. The chapter examines areas important to evaluate in addition to the typical components of program evaluation.

Chapter 10 provides an overview of the purpose and types of evaluation used in nursing simulation programs, including the numerous constructs that should be evaluated. Three types of evaluation (formative, summative, and high-stakes) are reviewed, and various data collection methods for use in simulation are presented with their challenges and strengths. Several categories of evaluation instruments exist, and the choice of which to use should align with the type of evaluation, learning objectives, and level of the learner. Accreditation is the next level of achievement for simulation programs that can show excellent outcomes as a result of their evaluation. Examples of the types of accreditation, the associated benefits, and program activities leading up to accreditation are presented in the chapter.

Effective practice-based education programs have much in common with the development and evaluation of academic nursing education programs. These programs are often based on assessed gaps in practice or requests from stakeholders in the organization. Nursing Professional Development (NPD) practitioners design and evaluate educational activities to address practice gaps for the identified target audience and improve providers' knowledge and skills. Chapter 11 provides an overview of the NPD role, describes types of practice-based education programs, discusses alignment with the NPD Scope and Standards of Practice competencies to demonstrate program evaluation, describes the Kirkpatrick model commonly used for program evaluation, and identifies common barriers to evaluating education programs in practice settings.

Thank you to the NLN for identifying the need for a second edition of this book to reflect the many changes that are occurring in nursing education that impact evaluation. The chapter authors deserve a special acknowledgement for sharing their expertise, helpful tips, and sample materials with readers, and for their enthusiasm about this book. We hope that you find the book valuable as you engage in evaluation of your nursing program.

Marilyn H. Oermann, PhD, RN, FAAN, ANEF
Thelma M. Ingles Professor of Nursing
Director of Educational Research
Duke University School of Nursing
Durham, North Carolina

Contents

List of Figures, Tables, and Boxes

LIST OF BOXES

1

Program Evaluation: What Is It?

Marilyn H. Oermann, PhD, RN, FAAN, ANEF

Program evaluation is a systematic process of collecting data for making decisions about a nursing program and judging its value. Evaluation is essential
to identify needs within the school, provide feedback while an educational program is
being developed, and establish the program's effectiveness and competencies of graduates following its completion. With evaluation that is done continuously, faculty, administrators, and other stakeholders learn what is working well in their nursing program and
where changes are needed to improve quality and outcomes. This chapter provides
an overview of program evaluation, beginning with the definitions of related concepts.

ASSESSMENT, EVALUATION, AND MEASUREMENT

Evaluation is essential for determining the effectiveness of the nursing program as a
whole and for individual courses and experiences within the program; for promoting
students' learning and professional development; and preparing them for future roles.
Evaluation allows faculty, administrators, and other stakeholders—people or groups
invested in the program—to systematically collect data and use those data for making
informed decisions that will improve program quality. Without evaluation, decisions may
be made based on tradition or what individuals and groups *think* will work best. With the
high cost of nursing education, and limited time for students to acquire the knowledge
and competencies they need for practice, decisions about the curriculum, instruction,
students, faculty, resources, and other areas need to be made carefully and based on
sound information.

Evaluation is integral to developing and maintaining a high-quality nursing program.
It cannot be done only for accreditation: evaluation should be part of the culture of the
school of nursing and done routinely when faculty, administrators, and others need
to make educational decisions. Evaluation provides the information for making those
decisions.

Terms such as assessment, evaluation, and measurement are sometimes used inter-
changeably, but there are differences that readers should be aware of. Assessment is
the process of obtaining information to use for making educational decisions (Brookhart &
Nitko, 2019; Oermann & Gaberson, 2021). Assessment in program evaluation is the collection

of aggregated data to determine if program and student learning outcomes, and other program goals, are in the process of being achieved or were achieved. In assessment, the educator collects information from various sources (Kane & Wools, 2020). Many strategies are available for collecting information related to an educational program including surveys of students, faculty, and other stakeholders; tests; focus groups; interviews; observations; rating scales; e-portfolios; and analyses of end-of-program projects, among others. The type of strategy needs to be appropriate for the purposes of the evaluation, and questions answered so as to provide the "right" information.

Evaluation is the process of making a judgment about the quality of a student's performance or the product being evaluated based on the information that was collected by the evaluator. Answering questions such as: How *well* did students perform on the comprehensive tests prior to and following the course revision?; What is the *effectiveness* of the on-campus intensive experience in developing students' competencies in interprofessional collaboration?; and How *satisfied* are students with the program? requires a value judgment. While assessment is the process of obtaining information, when judgments are made about quality, value, and worth, the process has extended to evaluation.

Measurement is not the same as assessment or evaluation. Measurement involves using scores or numbers to represent an outcome or characteristic. Mean scores on a survey of a course or program, test scores, and scales that indicate the quality of a student's performance in a skills laboratory are examples of measurements.

In this book, we use the term *evaluation* broadly to include information collected in an assessment of the program and the resulting judgments of quality. Those judgments lead faculty, administrators, and other stakeholders to decisions about needed improvements in the program or to maintain the program as is.

PURPOSES OF PROGRAM EVALUATION

There are many reasons to engage in program evaluation. All too often faculty and administrators think of program evaluation in terms of accreditation. While one of the purposes of program evaluation is to confirm that accreditation standards are met, this is only one purpose.

Through program evaluation, faculty can determine if students are achieving the outcomes of the program and the intended competencies. Assessment and evaluation are essential components of nursing courses, but program evaluation examines students' achievement and professional development across courses as they progress through the nursing program.

Program evaluation enables schools of nursing to identify needs within the school, the institution in which it is housed, and the community. Using this information, faculty and administrators may decide to develop a new course or program, revise current ones, begin or continue an initiative in the school, vary instructional methods, seek new clinical sites, or develop new resources, among others.

Program evaluation also provides data for modifying processes to improve efficiency and better meet student and other stakeholder needs. The information obtained through an evaluation can help faculty and administrators examine day-to-day processes in the program to assess if they are working well and to identify areas and practices in need of improvement. Questions such as, Is the clinical placement process effective, and what issues occur with arranging placements for students?, can be answered through a systematic evaluation, uncovering issues and leading to recommendations to improve processes.

Internal and External Evaluation Focus

Another way to think about the purposes of program evaluation is that they can be internal or external. Evaluation for internal purposes is not required by an accrediting body but is done within the school to answer questions of faculty, administrators, and others about various aspects of the program. Surveying students about their satisfaction with the simulation laboratory and adjunct faculty about the value of their orientation are examples of program evaluation done for internal reasons. Typically the goal of these evaluations is to make program improvements.

In contrast, external reasons are to verify that the nursing program meets the requirements and standards of the parent institution within which it is housed, the state board of nursing, and national nursing accrediting bodies. Institutions are accredited by regional accrediting agencies, such as the Southern Association of Colleges and Schools Commission on Colleges, which accredits degree-granting institutions in the Southern states. Accreditation at the institutional level documents that the community college, college, or university in which the nursing program is housed meets the standards of the accrediting agency. Program evaluation provides data about the nursing unit as part of the institution's accreditation. The evaluation process also verifies that a program meets state board of nursing requirements as an approved program within the state and the standards for nursing program accreditation through the Commission for Nursing Education Accreditation, Commission on Collegiate Nursing Education, and Accreditation Commission for Education in Nursing.

Formative and Summative Evaluation

Program evaluation is not only done at the end, when the program is completed, but also during its development to answer specific evaluation questions and identify where revisions are needed. The formative evaluation examines the program and its components while they are being developed and implemented. Formative data are used by faculty and administrators to identify and address issues and areas of the program needing further development. An example of a question asked during formative evaluation is: Is the integration of mental health concepts in the courses being implemented as intended?

Summative evaluation provides evidence of the effectiveness of the program and extent of outcomes achieved by students and graduates. This type of evaluation is used mainly for determining the quality of the program and whether students have achieved program outcomes and intended competencies. Summative evaluation takes place after the program is completed and implemented. Examples of questions for guiding summative evaluation are: Have students achieved the outcomes of the program? Can they perform competencies essential for entry into practice? What are the costs of a specific major or program offered by the school of nursing? Data from summative evaluation not only determine outcomes but also provide information for subsequent program improvement. Typically, summative data include information such as student scores on standardized tests, scores on end-of-program surveys, National Council Licensure Examination (NCLEX) and certification first-time pass rates, employment rates, and similar measures. Interviews and focus groups with stakeholders also may serve as summative data if the questions are intended to learn about participant responses to different experiences in the program and outcomes that have been achieved.

The differences between formative and summative evaluation relate to the use of the assessment data. When the information is used to provide feedback, the role is formative; when it is used for judgments about achievement, quality, or worth, the role is summative. Recently, views about formative and summative have shifted toward assessment for learning (formative) and assessment of learning (summative) (Kinnear et al., 2021; Oermann, 2022).

PROGRAM EVALUATION MODELS

There are many models, theories, and perspectives of program evaluation. Some commonly used models, summarized in this section of the chapter, are Context, Input, Process, Product (CIPP); logic; and Kirkpatrick's four-level. An evaluation also may focus on the processes or implementation of the program: is it being implemented as intended? Is the program meeting standards and expectations of stakeholders? Or, the evaluation may measure the impact of a program in meeting health care needs and accomplishing other goals, program outcomes, and costs-benefits. The model used to guide the program evaluation should answer the questions raised by educators, administrators, and other stakeholders about the program, and should provide the data needed to make informed decisions.

CIPP Model

Decision-oriented models provide information to educators for program improvement. An example of a decision-oriented model is the CIPP model (Stufflebeam & Zhang, 2017). This model includes an evaluation of each of its four components: context, input, process, and product. Evaluation that focuses on context is generally done when a new program is being planned or a program needs to be modified (Frye & Hemmer, 2012). Data for this component are often collected by reviewing program materials, analyzing demographic data and future trends, conducting surveys, and interviewing stakeholders. Input evaluation focuses on budgets, resources, and competing priorities of the setting to determine the best approaches to use after considering potential approaches. Data for this type of evaluation are often obtained through literature reviews, analyzing similar exemplary programs, and consulting with experts (Frye & Hemmer, 2012). In process evaluation, educators assess the implementation of the program and providing feedback to guide revisions. Is the program being implemented as planned? Information might be collected by observing students, faculty, and other aspects of the program; reviewing program materials; and interviewing stakeholders. In the CIPP model, product evaluation assesses program outcomes using surveys, such as exit surveys, studies of outcomes, tests, and interviews.

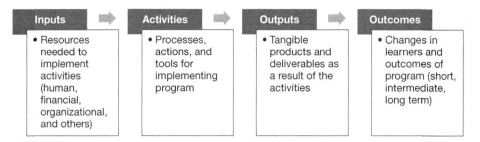

Inputs	⇒	Activities	⇒	Outputs	⇒	Outcomes
• Resources needed to implement activities (human, financial, organizational, and others)		• Processes, actions, and tools for implementing program		• Tangible products and deliverables as a result of the activities		• Changes in learners and outcomes of program (short, intermediate, long term)

FIGURE 1.1 Logic model.

Logic Model

For some types of program evaluation, a logic model is most appropriate (Fig. 1.1). While this model is often developed for program planning, it also can be used for evaluating a program. A logic model is a graphic depiction that presents the relationships among:

> Inputs (resources including human, financial, organizational, and others).
> Activities (processes, actions, and tools for implementing the program and accomplishing the intended program changes or results).
> Outputs (tangible products and deliverables that result from the activities).
> Outcomes (changes in learner knowledge, skills, and behaviors, and short-term, intermediate, and long-term outcomes of a program.
(Centers for Disease Control and Prevention, Program Performance and Evaluation Office, 2018)

A logic model is developed starting with the program's intended outcomes (short-term, intermediate, and long-term) and then moving from the right-hand side to the left (Idzik et al., 2021). After identifying the desired outcomes or goals, the evaluator works backward—right to left, from outcomes to inputs—to determine the outputs or tangible products and deliverables that are needed for these outcomes, then the activities to be done, and then the essential inputs or resources.

There are many variations of the logic model, but, in general, this model provides a systematic way to view the relationships among the resources for offering the program, activities to be done, and anticipated changes or outcomes. Figure 1.2 provides an example of a logic model for evaluating an academic-practice partnership in nursing. Another example is available on the CDC website (https://www.cdc.gov/tb/programs/evaluation/Logic_Model.html). Many resources are available on the Internet for developing a logic model for program planning and evaluation.

Kirkpatrick's Model

Kirkpatrick's four-level model is used widely for evaluating learner outcomes. In this model, there are four levels of outcomes to be evaluated:

1. Reaction: satisfaction of learners with the program (what program participants thought about the program).

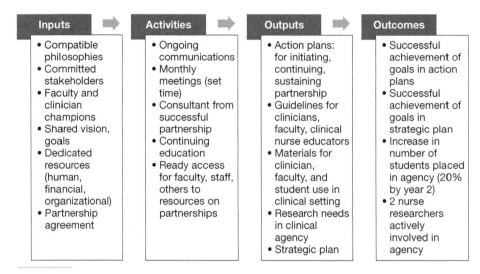

FIGURE 1.2 Example of a logic model for evaluating academic-practice partnership.

2. Learning: gains in knowledge, skills, and attitudes as a result of the education or specific training (what participants learned from the program).

3. Behavior: changes in learners' behaviors.

4. Results: long-term results or outcomes.

    (Kirkpatrick & Kirkpatrick, 2015)

Using Kirkpatrick's model helps focus the evaluation on more than learners' satisfaction with and perceptions of the program, and their knowledge and skills. This model, while easy to understand and use, however, focuses on learner-related outcomes and does not provide for a comprehensive evaluation of an educational program.

STEPS IN PROGRAM EVALUATION

While there are many models, theories, and perspectives of program evaluation, one constant across all of them is that program evaluation is a systematic and planned process. This is an important concept because the evaluation needs to provide the "right" information to make decisions about the program and to answer educator, administrator, and other stakeholder questions.

Identify Purpose of Evaluation

The evaluation process begins by identifying its purpose (Box 1.1). The evaluation may be comprehensive and broad, for example, evaluating outcomes of the program, or narrow in scope, such as determining the effectiveness of a peer tutoring program. The purpose of the evaluation and scope also influence the extent of resources (time, costs) needed to complete the evaluation. An evaluation that is narrow and more focused generally requires less time and fewer resources.

BOX 1.1

Steps in Program Evaluation

1. Identify purpose of the evaluation.
2. Develop questions to be answered through evaluation.
3. Design the evaluation.
4. Collect and analyze the evaluation data.
5. Report findings and use for program improvement, if indicated.

Develop Questions to be Answered through Evaluation

Considering the purpose of the evaluation, the next step is to identify the questions to be answered. An example of a question related to program outcomes is: What is the first-time pass rate on the NCLEX for graduates of the BSN program? To examine the effectiveness of the tutoring program, a question might be: Do students who participate in peer tutoring achieve passing grades in their pathophysiology course and are they satisfied with the tutoring program? The evaluation is designed and implemented to answer those questions. The questions not only provide the starting point for a program evaluation, but also can be used as organizing themes for the evaluation (Rossi, Lipsey, & Henry, 2019).

Design the Evaluation

The evaluation questions guide the design of the evaluation and the types of data collected. This is the step in which the faculty, administrators, or other evaluators identify the information needed to answer their questions. Some of the data may be available currently in the program; if not, surveys, tools, and other strategies will need to be identified to provide the essential data. This step in the evaluation process also includes deciding on the time frame for data collection. For example, to assess the effectiveness of the peer tutoring program intended to promote success in the pathophysiology course, grades in the course and findings on a survey of students' satisfaction with the tutoring would be examined at the end of the course. These data might be collected only at this one point in time. However, to assess students' perceptions of their achievement of program outcomes and satisfaction with the program, data might be collected at the end of the program through an exit survey, and from alumni one year post graduation.

Collect and Analyze Evaluation Data

The next step is to collect and analyze the data. The evaluation plan should specify the expected levels of performance or benchmarks to be met. These are essential for interpreting the data. For example, for the question on first-time NCLEX pass rate, the expected level of performance might be for 90% of graduates to pass the NCLEX the first time taken. For peer tutoring, the expected level might be that 95% of the students who complete all tutoring sessions pass the pathophysiology course, and 85% report satisfaction with the tutoring on a survey.

Report Findings and Use for Program Improvement, if Indicated

The findings from the evaluation should be communicated to faculty, administrators, and others for making decisions about the program. Individuals and groups involved in the evaluation should continually review the data to determine if changes or other actions are indicated. Opsahl and Horton-Deutsch (2019) developed a nursing program dashboard that conveys the results of the evaluation in a user-friendly format, allowing stakeholders to continually monitor nursing program quality and examine longitudinal program trends. Data also might be shared on the intranet, in meetings with stakeholders, through narrative summaries, and by other strategies. Consideration should be given to how frequently to disseminate the results to faculty, administrators, and other stakeholders.

Summary

Program evaluation is a systematic process of collecting information about a nursing program for making informed decisions. Through evaluation, faculty, administrators, and others can judge the quality, value, and worth of the program and its many components. Evaluation is essential to identify needs within the school, provide feedback while a program is being developed, and establish the program's effectiveness following its completion. With evaluation that is done continuously, faculty, administrators, and other stakeholders learn what is working well in their nursing program and where changes are needed to improve quality.

References

Brookhart, S. M., & Nitko, A. J. (2019). *Educational assessment of students.* (9th ed.). Pearson Education.

Centers for Disease Control and Prevention Program. Performance and Evaluation Office. (2018). *Program evaluation framework checklist for step 2: Describe the program.* Accessed June 7, 2022. https://www.cdc.gov/eval/steps/step2/index.htm

Frye, A. W., & Hemmer, P. A. (2012). Program evaluation models and related theories: AMEE Guide No. 67. *Medical Teacher, 34*(5), e288–e299. https://doi.org/10.3109/0142159X.2012.668637

Idzik, S., Buckley, K., Bindon, S., Gorschboth, S., Hammersla, M., Windemuth, B., & Bingham, D. (2021). Lessons learned using logic models to design and guide DNP projects. *Nurse Educator, 46*(5), E127–E131. https://doi.org/10.1097/nne.0000000000001025

Kane, M. T., & Wools, S. (2020). Perspectives on the validity of classroom assessments. In S. M. Brookhart & J. H. McMillan (Eds.), *Classroom assessment and educational measurement* (pp. 11–26). Routledge.

Kinnear, B., Warm, E. J., Caretta-Weyer, H., Holmboe, E. S., Turner, D. A., van der Vleuten, C., & Schumacher, D. J. (2021). Entrustment unpacked: Aligning purposes, stakes, and processes to enhance learner assessment. *Academic Medicine, 96*(7S), S56–S63. doi: 10.1097/ACM.0000000000004108

Kirkpatrick, J., & Kirkpatrick, W. (2015). *An introduction to the new world Kirkpatrick® model*. Kirkpatrick Partners.

Oermann, M. H. (2022). Some principles to guide assessment of competencies. *Nurse Educator, 47*(1), 1. https://doi.org/10.1097/nne.0000000000001143

Oermann, M. H., & Gaberson, K. B. (2021). *Evaluation and testing in nursing education.* (6th ed.). Springer.

Opsahl, A., & Horton-Deutsch, S. (2019). A nursing dashboard to communicate the evaluation of program outcomes. *Nurse Educator, 44*(6), 326–329. doi: 10.1097/NNE.0000000000000632

Rossi, P. H., Lipsey, M. W., & Henry, G. T. (2019). *Evaluation: A systematic approach.* (8th ed.). SAGE Publications.

Stufflebeam, D. L., & Zhang, G. (2017). *The CIPP evaluation model: How to evaluate for improvement and accountability*. Guilford Press.

2

Curriculum Evaluation

Theresa M. "Terry" Valiga, EdD, RN, CNE, FAAN, ANEF
Jacquelyn McMillian-Bohler, PhD, CNM, CNE

F aculty in schools of nursing often spend a great deal of time designing a curriculum that provides students with an organized approach to learning a new nursing role, implementing that curriculum in ways that engage the learner and effectively employ creative strategies, and evaluating what students have learned as a result of those experiences. However, efforts to evaluate the entire curriculum often are overlooked, not approached in a systematic way, undocumented, and incomplete. This chapter addresses the purposes of and ways to approach curriculum evaluation that relates this activity to the evaluation of an overall program, and clarifies the role of faculty in the curriculum development, evaluation, and revision processes.

CURRICULUM DEVELOPMENT AND EVALUATION: WHY

Often when we think of "curriculum," we think of a collection of courses, the rigid sequencing of courses, the content to be covered, the required prerequisites, the hours:credit ratios, and even the plan to achieve desired licensing or certification examination results. But a curriculum is much more than these things. In essence, the curriculum is a *gestalt* that incorporates hoped-for, as well as unanticipated, outcomes; the variety of experiences designed to enhance student learning; the assessment and evaluation methods used; the diverse pedagogical perspectives of faculty; and the relationships between and among students and teachers. It also has been referred to as stories to be heard (Ironside, 2004; Tanner, 2004), a culture of excellence, the full engagement of participants in learning and growing, the complex and dynamic connections among learning experiences, the material to be learned, and the values to be reflected upon.

When evaluating a curriculum, it is not enough to focus only on student evaluations of courses or teachers, peer review of a teaching session or an online course, graduation rates, or licensure or certification examination pass rates. Instead, all components of the curriculum need to be examined for the extent to which they are relevant, effective, reflective of professional standards and current concerns, and critical to developing graduates who can thrive in today's complex, uncertain, ambiguous, technology-rich, ever-changing health care environment and who can shape the future of health care and the nursing profession. *This* is the purpose of curriculum evaluation.

CURRICULUM EVALUATION AND PROGRAM EVALUATION: RELATED BUT DIFFERENT

Program evaluation should address all the elements needed to offer a quality nursing program and prepare graduates for practice. Those elements are reflected in the standards used by nursing's accreditation bodies (Accreditation Commission for Education in Nursing, 2020; Commission on Collegiate Nursing Education, 2018; National League for Nursing [NLN] Commission for Nursing Education Accreditation, 2018) and the regulations established by the relevant State Board of Nursing. Such standards address mission, governance, resources, program outcomes, faculty, students, curriculum, teaching/learning practices, and program effectiveness.

In addition, for those schools aiming beyond minimum standards and toward a level of excellence, the NLN's *Hallmarks of Excellence in Nursing Education Model* (2020) identified eight hallmarks that guide schools toward distinction: engaged students; diverse, well-prepared faculty; a culture of continuous quality improvement; innovative, evidence-based curriculum; innovative, evidence-based approaches to facilitate and evaluate learning; resources to support program goal attainment; commitment to pedagogical scholarship; and effective institutional and professional leadership. The Curriculum section of that document notes the following hallmarks:

➤ The curriculum is designed to help students achieve stated program outcomes, reflects current societal and health care trends and issues, and is responsive to change and evolving societal needs. The curriculum also embeds evidence-based information, reflects research findings and innovative practices, attends to the evolving role of the nurse in a variety of settings, is flexible and innovative, and incorporates local, national, and global perspectives.

➤ The curriculum provides learning activities that enhance students' abilities to think critically, reflect thoughtfully, and provide culturally sensitive, evidence-based nursing care to diverse populations.

➤ The curriculum emphasizes students' values development, identity formation, caring for self, commitment to lifelong learning, critical thinking, ethical and evidence-based practice, and creativity.

➤ The curriculum provides learning experiences that prepare graduates to assume roles that are essential to quality nursing practice, including, but not limited to, roles of care provider, advocate for those in need, teacher, communicator, change agent, care coordinator, member of intra- and interprofessional teams, user of information technology, collaborator, decision-maker, leader, and evolving scholar.

➤ The curriculum provides learning experiences that support evidence-based practice, interprofessional approaches to care, student achievement of clinical competence, and, as appropriate, competence in a specialty role.

Using these hallmarks and the indicators outlined for each—all of which are discussed extensively by Adams and Valiga (2021)—challenges faculty to think deeply about what they are trying to accomplish through their curriculum and can serve as an additional set of expectations to use for curriculum evaluation. Whatever the standards or indicators used, faculty should "set the bar high" and not settle for mediocrity. The preparation of graduates for the significant roles they will have in the future requires that faculty strive for excellence and not be satisfied with the status quo or merely doing things the way they have always been done.

Thus, ongoing evaluation of an overall program requires a careful look at many elements, one of which is the curriculum. It is clear that to implement the curriculum, well-prepared faculty are needed, as are administrative support and resources that are adequate and of high-quality. Curriculum evaluation, therefore, cannot be complete unless many of these components are addressed. Program evaluation is a larger concept that subsumes curriculum evaluation, which is the focus of this chapter.

WHAT CURRICULUM COMPONENTS SHOULD BE EVALUATED AND WHEN?

What are the essential components that need to be studied to determine the relevance and effectiveness of the curriculum? A curriculum evaluation should include a review of the program philosophy, conceptual framework, program outcomes, level outcomes, design of the curriculum (i.e., sequencing of courses), teaching strategies, evaluation methods, and the community partners who support learners. Although the elements of a comprehensive curriculum review are fixed, the timeline for reviewing various components will vary.

Philosophy

The school's philosophy is an expression of the values and beliefs of the faculty about human beings, society/context/environment, health/health care, nursing/nurses, and education/teaching-learning. It is important that faculty regularly review the philosophy to reflect on whether the beliefs expressed in it remain current, and to determine the extent to which the expressed beliefs and values truly guide decisions and day-to-day actions. For example, the philosophy may indicate that the faculty support individualized, student-centered learning; on reflection, however, faculty may realize that there is little or no opportunity throughout the curriculum for students to follow their individualized passions, learn in ways that are most effective for them, or do anything other than follow the teacher-directed path. Such a realization should lead faculty to reflect on how deeply this value is held and what they might do differently to "make it come alive" and be more than mere words on a page.

Additionally, the philosophy may assert values related to diversity, equity, and inclusion, as well as a recognition that individuals prefer to learn in different ways, at different times, and with different resources. However, if all students are expected to do the same thing in the same way at the same time, if lecture is the only teaching strategy used, or if multiple-choice tests are the only evaluation method, one must wonder whether such philosophical statements are genuine and truly guide action. Further examples of implications of statements in the philosophy provide additional areas for reflection (Valiga, 2020).

Values and beliefs are not expected to change dramatically in a short period of time, so it is not necessary to engage in deep reflection and invite possible major revisions of the philosophy every semester or on an annual basis; instead, this might be an activity that is undertaken with seriousness every 5 to 6 years. However, programs may find it beneficial to review and discuss the school's philosophy annually to ensure that it guides student-teacher relationships, as well as day-to-day teaching practices.

Conceptual Framework

Although most schools do not use a single theory—nursing or otherwise—as the framework for the curriculum, there needs to be some type of "umbrella" that guides faculty in writing program outcomes, designing the learning sequence, and deciding where to place emphases. The concepts evident in this "umbrella" may be *pervasive* (i.e., consistently addressed, regardless of where students are in the program), or they may be *progressive* in nature (i.e., developed in increasing depth and complexity from the beginning to the end of the program). Regardless of the nature of a particular concept, it is essential that the key concepts that undergird the entire curriculum be relevant, clearly defined, and understood by all. As a result of ongoing environmental scanning, stakeholder feedback, and literature review, it becomes increasingly clear that today's nursing curricula must help students develop the understandings, skills, and values needed to function effectively as a professional. This includes engaging effectively in person-centered, collaborative practice that is based on evidence; exhibiting a spirit of inquiry; engaging in lifelong learning and professional development; and acting as a leader when needed.

Similar to the values expressed in the philosophy, the concepts that serve as the framework for the curriculum are not likely to change often, but it is essential that faculty regularly reflect on whether they are congruent with current discussions about health, health care, and nursing practice. A review of the conceptual framework can occur at the same time as the review of the philosophy, and that is every 5 to 6 years.

Program Outcomes

Program outcomes are statements of student achievement, specifying what they should know, be able to do, and value or appreciate upon completion of the program. They are important because they allow for accountability, serve as a basis for evaluation of the effectiveness of the program, are essential for accreditation requirements, clarify what employers should expect, and give direction to future program planning.

Since the most central indication of academic quality is student learning, program outcomes must be *student-focused*. Additionally, because they reflect the totality of student achievement as the result of the entire course of study, program outcomes should be *complex* and *multifaceted*.

When evaluating program outcomes, faculty should consider the clarity with which they have defined the qualities and characteristics of graduates on completion of the program, the realities of today's practice arenas, whether they address preparing graduates for an unknown future and a lifetime career, the values expressed in the school's philosophy, the concepts articulated in the framework, and new insights about learning. Consideration also should be given to characteristics of the school's unique student body, the time available to realistically achieve each outcome, and the resources available to achieve the stated ends. Finally, program outcomes should use unambiguous language and be measurable; however, it is important to remember that multiple means to measure achievement of the outcomes is essential in light of their complexity and multifaceted nature.

Because program outcomes are key to determining how the curriculum will be designed and implemented, it is important to review them regularly. Additionally, it may be beneficial to involve practice partners and other community stakeholders in establishing and revising program outcomes to ensure those outcomes are consistent with current and evolving industry needs. A careful review every 2 to 3 years may be in order to ensure that the outcomes remain relevant and that all faculty understand them in the same way. While words can be changed to clarify meaning, a major overhaul of program outcomes is warranted only when faculty are committed to a thorough review of the entire curriculum and prepared to make major revisions as needed.

Level Outcomes

Level outcomes can be thought of as the "signposts" along the journey to the overall program outcomes. A school may define a "level" in any number of ways (e.g., by academic year or by semester), but it is important to remember that the "cluster" of courses included in a level should have some consistency among them. For example, a school may define Level I as the first of a six-semester baccalaureate program, where the focus is on laying a foundation related to the profession of nursing, basic knowledge and skills, and wellness. Level II might include semesters two, three, and four of nursing courses, where the focus is on caring for different patient populations (e.g., children, pregnant women, and the elderly) and the nursing care needed to help them maintain or regain health. Finally, Level III might include the final two semesters of the program, which focus on caring for patients with complex health care needs, collaborating with the interprofessional team, functioning as a leader, and making the transition from the role of student to that of graduate nurse.

Level outcomes, then, should define the expected accomplishments of students as a result of the learning experiences in the cluster of courses at a given level; thus, they complement but are different from individual course objectives. Additionally, they should show increasing complexity of student knowledge, skills, and values as the student moves from one level to the next.

When evaluating a program's level outcomes, faculty should look for clarity, congruence with the program outcomes, and whether they are realistic, given the course experiences included in a particular level. If there is a mismatch between course experiences and level outcomes, faculty need to decide (a) if the courses are not designed well enough to help students achieve the level outcomes or (b) if the stated level outcomes are unrealistic. Faculty also should examine whether the level outcomes truly progress in complexity, serve to illustrate the unique focus of each level and how each level builds on the previous one, and whether all are leading toward accomplishment of the program outcomes.

As was noted for program outcomes, analysis and reflection of level outcomes can be undertaken every 2 to 3 years, with minor changes for clarification. Major revisions, though, should be avoided until faculty are committed to a thorough review of the curriculum and prepared to make major changes as needed.

Curriculum Design

The curriculum design is the sequence in which students take courses in a variety of areas — nursing; foundational physical, social, and behavioral sciences; the liberal arts; and electives. To evaluate the design, faculty need to assess the extent to which students have the necessary foundation (i.e., what they have learned in foundational or prerequisite courses) on which to build nursing courses (Valiga, 2015); the degree of flexibility in the course of study; the logical flow of course experiences; the extent to which the values expressed in the philosophy and concepts articulated in the framework are evident; and the extent to which the "collection" of courses in any given semester are aligned with the level and ultimately the program outcomes. Ongoing reviews of course evaluations are likely to give clues to weaknesses in the curriculum design; however, to avoid significant disruptions for the learners, major curriculum design changes should be undertaken only after program and level outcomes have been reviewed carefully.

Courses

Summative evaluation of courses often is done only through student feedback at the end of the term and using standardized forms. While such an approach is valuable, it is not sufficient. Course evaluations also should address whether students came into the course with the necessary foundation, the degree to which faculty built on or repeated foundational knowledge, the depth of student learning, and the extent to which students *and* faculty believe the foundation needed to be successful in subsequent courses has been built. Additionally, courses should be evaluated in terms of the effectiveness of methods and resources used in the course (e.g., case studies, team-based learning, and textbooks) in facilitating learning, and the appropriateness of assessment and evaluation methods used in the course to judge student attainment of the objectives. Finally, consideration should be given to the nature of the learning environment that existed in the course, ways in which student/student and student/teacher interactions were encouraged, and the degree to which the learning needs of the diverse student population were met.

Summative evaluation of courses is helpful, but faculty also should consider formative evaluation of courses. Gathering information about the clarity of learning objectives, effectiveness of strategies used to facilitate and methods used to assess learning, nature of the learning environment, relationships among students and faculty, and other elements while the course is in process and some changes can be made "before it's too late" also is helpful to ensure positive learning experiences.

In addition to evaluating courses—as well as the Teaching/Learning Strategies and Assessment/Evaluation Methods used in them—faculty also need to examine whether biases are built into courses. Bias within courses and/or the overall curriculum can introduce and reinforce stereotypes, which then perpetuate health disparities and ultimately impact patient outcomes negatively (Sherman et al., 2019). Additionally, exposure to bias can cause some learners to feel isolated, ashamed, disillusioned, or angry, all of which create barriers to learning. To address bias within courses and the overall curriculum, faculty should first identify and reflect on their beliefs about race, gender, religion, ability, age, sexual orientation, socioeconomic status, immigration status, and weight. Then, they should use this "lens" to critically evaluate all aspects of the curriculum and be honest with themselves as they do so, since bias often is implicit and unconsciously committed. Using a structured process, or rubric, to evaluate courses and the overall curriculum for bias can ensure an effective review. Examples of such comprehensive models include (a) *Assessing Bias in Standards & Curricular Materials Tool* (Coomer et al., 2017) and (b) *Inclusive and Bias-Free Checklist,* adapted by the Northwestern University Feinberg School of Medicine (2021) from a tool created by Curaso Brown.

While certain elements of courses, for example, teaching strategies, evaluation methods, and resources used, should be reviewed regularly, care needs to be taken when considering revisions to course objectives, prerequisites, course credits, and similar components. Since these latter elements are highly dependent on and integral to other curriculum components, such as framework, program and level outcomes, and design, they should be changed only as part of "big picture" revisions.

Teaching/Learning Strategies

The primary considerations that should be given when evaluating the teaching and learning strategies used in a course, are whether they effectively facilitate student learning and the degree to which they engage students as active learners. Faculty also should ensure that the strategies used are based on evidence, and are designed and implemented in accord with best practices.

Whether students liked using case studies, brainstorming, or concept maps is helpful to know, but the more important question addresses the extent to which these approaches helped them learn and achieve course objectives. Additionally, while it is important to know if faculty liked teaching online or using certain teaching strategies, it is critical to determine if the course was well organized, made reasonable expectations of students, ensured that students were adequately prepared to engage in specific learning activities, and was implemented effectively.

Such evaluations are ongoing and should be done each time a course is taught. In this way, faculty can be assured that teaching/learning practices are informed by pedagogical research and are effective in facilitating learning for diverse and changing student populations.

Assessment/Evaluation Methods

Similar to evaluating teaching/learning strategies, faculty need to evaluate the effectiveness of the methods used in the course to determine student achievement of course objectives. Questions should be raised about the fairness of methods, the reasonableness of how each is weighted when calculating the course grade, variety of approaches used, and rationale for each method. Each learning objective should have an evaluation strategy, but it is important to keep in mind that a single evaluation method may be aligned with more than one objective. In addition, faculty should ensure that each of the domains of learning—cognitive, psychomotor, and affective—appropriate to the course are assessed. For example, if only multiple-choice tests are used to assess student learning, does that convey a message to students that only cognitive knowledge is important?

Assessment/evaluation methods also should focus on students' writing, speaking, presentation, and leadership skills; their ability to manage uncertainty and ambiguity; the effectiveness of their interactions with others (patients, peers, nurses in clinical settings, members of the health care team); the clarity and strength of their individual values; and an understanding of how personal values influence their behaviors. Faculty may find that there is a need to identify some courses as writing-intensive so that students are challenged to develop these skills throughout the program. Or they may determine that certain courses should include professional presentations for students to get feedback on their ability to present in an organized fashion, argue convincingly, respond to questions from others, "think on their feet," and speak in an articulate manner. Alternatively, some assessment/evaluation methods will need to be directly observed in a clinical or simulation experience. Thus, evaluation of assessment/evaluation methods involve more than merely doing item analyses on a multiple-choice test to determine if a question is a good one or not.

Like the teaching/learning strategies used, the methods used to assess/evaluate learning need to be evaluated on an ongoing basis, particularly as pedagogical research informs faculty of the effectiveness of various methods to assess and evaluate learning. Evaluation of methods used to assess learning, therefore, should occur each time a course is taught.

Resources and Partnerships

The final curriculum component to be evaluated relates to the resources available to support course implementation and student achievement of course objectives and, ultimately, level and program outcomes. Such resources include physical space, online learning management systems, laboratory equipment and supplies, library resources, clinical facilities, counseling resources, writing skills resources, and faculty qualifications and teaching abilities. It also is important to reflect on the nature of partnerships that have been established with various inpatient clinical units, outpatient clinics, home care agencies, community agencies, and others. A "breakdown" in any of these areas can sorely undermine the effectiveness of a curriculum, so they must be attended to carefully, seriously, and regularly as part of curriculum evaluation.

A Summary of What and When to Evaluate

As noted, a curriculum is a gestalt that incorporates many aspects, and each one of those components needs to be evaluated to ensure the curriculum remains relevant and effective. Table 2.1 provides a summary of what should be evaluated, why it is important to evaluate each component, and ideas regarding how to do such evaluations. Similarly, Table 2.2 provides a summary of when each curriculum component should be evaluated.

TABLE 2.1

Summary of Elements of Curriculum Evaluation

What		Why	How
Philosophy	➤ Are the values and beliefs of the faculty about human beings, society/context/environment, health/healthcare, nurses/nursing, and education/teaching-learning reflected?	Clarifies the values and beliefs of the faculty that will influence decision-making and day-to-day practices	➤ Faculty retreat ➤ Survey
Conceptual Framework	➤ Are core curriculum concepts clearly defined? ➤ Is it congruent with the philosophy? ➤ Are the core concepts evident in the Program Outcomes?	Provides faculty with a guide for writing program outcomes, designing the learning sequence, and deciding where to place emphases in the curriculum	➤ Ask faculty to describe the meaning of each concept ➤ Ask students to describe/demonstrate the meaning of each concept ➤ Survey ➤ Faculty retreat
Program Outcomes	➤ Are they consistent with the philosophy and framework? ➤ Do they prepare students to take on the role they seek to assume? ➤ Can they be measured? ➤ Do they meet the needs of employers?	Clearly defines what students should know, be able to do, and value or appreciate upon completion of the program	➤ Feedback from employers ➤ Feedback from alumni ➤ Consultant review ➤ Review current literature
Level Outcomes	➤ Can they be assessed? ➤ Are they reasonable in light of student characteristics and available resources? ➤ Do they address all domains of learning (cognitive, psychomotor, and affective)?	Ensures clearly defined measures for the successful progress of students through the program	➤ Faculty retreat ➤ Consultant review ➤ Student feedback
Curriculum Design	➤ Are stated prerequisites appropriate and necessary to prepare students for the course? ➤ Is there internal consistency among all the courses? ➤ Is the course sequencing logical?	Ensures the curriculum has a consistent, organized, and logical design	➤ Student feedback ➤ Mapping ➤ Program catalog/syllabi ➤ Consultant review

TABLE 2.1		
Summary of Elements of Curriculum Evaluation *(Continued)*		
What	**Why**	**How**
Courses ➤ Do course objectives align with outcomes for the appropriate level? ➤ Do courses increase in complexity throughout the program? ➤ Does course content align with course objectives? ➤ Are there signs of implicit and explicit bias in the course design and/or implementation?	Evaluates the degree to which faculty build upon or repeat foundational knowledge, the depth of student learning, and the extent to which students and faculty believe the foundation needed to be successful in subsequent courses has been built	➤ Course evaluation form(s) ➤ Curriculum committee review ➤ Stakeholder advisory board input ➤ Student evaluations ➤ Syllabi review
Teaching & Learning Strategies ➤ Do they engage students and facilitate their learning? ➤ Are they reflective of evolving evidence and best practices? ➤ Are they varied to meet diverse student learning needs and preferences? ➤ Do they support inclusiveness and avoid implicit bias? ➤ Are they consistent with beliefs about teaching/learning expressed in the philosophy?	Evaluates the effectiveness of strategies to facilitate student learning and active engagement in the learning process	➤ Results of students' evaluations of teaching ➤ Review and reflection ➤ Course evaluation forms ➤ Consultant review ➤ Course or program committee reviews
Assessment & Evaluation Methods ➤ Are they fair/reasonable? ➤ Are they appropriate in light of stated learning objectives? ➤ Do they reflect all three domains of learning? ➤ Do they clearly assess students' achievement of course objectives and competencies? ➤ Do they support inclusiveness and avoid implicit bias?	Ensures assessment and evaluation methods effectively and appropriately assess student achievement of course objectives	➤ Item analyses ➤ Review of the literature ➤ Course evaluation forms ➤ Stakeholder feedback ➤ Performance on licensure examinations ➤ Test development committee analyses

(continued)

TABLE 2.1

Summary of Elements of Curriculum Evaluation *(Continued)*

What		Why	How
Resources & Partnerships	➤ Are they adequate to assist students in meeting program outcomes? ➤ Are graduates prepared for practice? ➤ Are clinical sites appropriate for learning outcomes and learners? ➤ Are clinical partners involved in curriculum design? ➤ Are the appropriate faculty teaching courses?	Ensures sufficient resources are available to support course implementation and student achievement of course objectives and, ultimately, level and program outcomes	➤ Feedback from clinical partners ➤ Alumni feedback ➤ Course evaluations ➤ Course reports

TABLE 2.2

Curriculum Evaluation Timeline

WHAT to Evaluate	WHEN to Evaluate
Philosophy	Every 5–6 years
Conceptual framework	Every 5–6 years
Program outcomes	Every 2–3 years Review when State Board of Nursing requirements or accreditation standards change significantly or when significant changes in nursing occur
Level outcomes	Every 2–3 years Any time program outcomes are revised
Curriculum design	Every 2–3 years Any time program and level outcomes are revised
Courses	Every time course is taught Consider formative evaluations while course is underway
Teaching/learning strategies	Every time course is taught Consider formative evaluations while course is underway
Evaluation/assessment methods	Every time course is taught Consider formative evaluations while course is underway
Partnerships and resources	Every time course is taught Formalized discussions with clinical partners annually

DATA COLLECTION STRATEGIES: HOW SHOULD FACULTY APPROACH CURRICULUM EVALUATION?

There is no "one and only one" or one "right" way to collect data about the effectiveness of the curriculum. Faculty, therefore, have the freedom to construct approaches that are workable for them and that will yield information to help them determine what to continue, what to modify, what to change dramatically, what to eliminate, and when a major curriculum revision is needed. Although certain aspects of curriculum evaluation can be assigned to a task force or committee, all faculty should be heavily involved in data collection and analysis processes. Additionally, curriculum evaluation data also should be collected from many stakeholders to ensure that the evaluation is comprehensive. Options for data collection about the curriculum are varied.

> **Plan annual retreats** that focus on a "deep dive" into all or part of the curriculum. For example, one year the focus might be on the constellation of courses in Level I where faculty look critically at the degree to which those courses are congruent with the school's philosophy and framework, the extent to which they align with the level outcomes, what the faculty teaching in subsequent courses says about the preparedness of students as they enter those upper-level courses, the effectiveness of any writing-intensive courses, the variety of teaching and learning strategies and assessment/evaluation methods used, what students said about their experiences, feedback from clinical staff who worked with students, student performance on tests and other measures of their learning, and so on. This 360-degree review of Level I would lead faculty to make recommendations about any changes that might be needed and what they would look for to determine if those changes were effective. In the following year, the same process could be applied to the constellation of courses in Level II and continue until data are collected on each level of the curriculum.

> **Use the Self-Assessment Checklist** developed by Adams and Valiga (2020, pp. 163–181) and based on the *Hallmarks of Excellence in Nursing Education* (NLN, 2020). Faculty might be asked to complete the checklist individually and then again in a retreat-like forum, compare their responses, discuss areas with widely divergent views, and determine what changes, if any, are needed to meet the hallmarks.

> **Invite an external curriculum expert** (from another part of the university or another school) to review the curriculum, examine the extent to which all components are internally consistent, and assess how the curriculum aligns with selected accreditation standards or other benchmarks. This individual could then engage in dialogue with faculty about areas of strength and concern, and how those areas of concern could be addressed.

> **Conduct focus groups or open dialogue** with clinical partners on a regular basis. Faculty should seek input on how graduates of their nursing program compare to graduates of other programs in terms of their ability to think critically, provide quality care, work collaboratively with others, and meet other expectations. This also would be an excellent opportunity to discuss the quality of students' clinical experiences, the supportiveness of clinical staff, the extent to which students and clinical instructors perceive that they are an integral part of the practice

environment, communication patterns, and other elements that impact the quality and effectiveness of student clinical experiences.

▸ **Critically reflect on the philosophy** to determine if the values expressed in it still reflect the thinking of the faculty. As mentioned, this might be done only every 5 to 6 years, but it is a step that should not be forgotten. One way to approach this analysis is to create a survey that asks faculty to examine each sentence in the philosophy and provide input on whether they think it continues to be accurate and essential, is important but does not need to be stated in the philosophy, is no longer congruent with current practice or trends, and so forth. Faculty also could be asked to share values that may be absent from the current document and should be added. A team could do an analysis of the survey results, share them with faculty as a whole or in small groups, discuss the findings, and make recommendations for changes that might be needed in the document.

▸ **Critically reflect on the framework** to determine if the key concepts on which the curriculum has been built remain relevant and if all concepts essential for contemporary nursing practice (e.g., interprofessional collaboration, evidence-based practice, patient-centered care, information management) are incorporated and fully developed. Such an analysis would be enhanced by careful environmental scanning, in which faculty have reviewed the essence of key documents, organizational recommendations, current literature, and input from stakeholders such as alumni and employers. The key points from these resources could be summarized and mapped against the existing curriculum concepts to identify areas of congruence and where the curriculum concepts might be deficient or inadequate considering today's environment and the yet-to-be-determined environment of the future.

▸ **Use a course report form** (see Fig. 2.1 for an example) each time a course is taught to document details of the course, what was effective, how students responded to various learning activities, what challenged the teacher, what resources were helpful and which were needed, what should be revised, etc. Course teams, program faculty, and/or curriculum committees can then review all course report forms to identify curriculum strengths, areas that need immediate attention, areas to consider for long-term revisions, patterns of concerns, and so on.

FACULTY ROLE IN CURRICULUM DEVELOPMENT, EVALUATION, AND REVISION PROCESSES

Once faculty have engaged in curriculum evaluation activities, they are challenged to reflect on what those data mean and the implications for curriculum refinement or a major revision. During this phase of curriculum development, faculty need to be willing to abandon "sacred cows" and accept that courses they have been teaching may need significant revision in terms of the objectives and focus, teaching/learning strategies, and/or evaluation methods.

Faculty may discover that the values expressed in the philosophy are not really guiding the design or implementation of the curriculum. Or they may unearth many disconnects among the various curriculum components. For example, concepts identified in the framework may be evident only in beginning courses but not integrated throughout the program, or concepts may be emphasized in final-semester courses that have not even been introduced previously. They may find that the curriculum is not effective in helping students develop their identities as nurses, nurse practitioners, or scholars. Interpreting the meaning of curriculum evaluation data also may highlight for faculty that the data are not completely informative because benchmarks for what is expected to be achieved have not been established.

Although it is possible that data from curriculum evaluation efforts reveal that everything is perfect and no revisions are needed, the greater likelihood is that a number of areas needing attention will be identified. Faculty should then weigh the significance of each area and its impact on preparing students effectively, and outline plans for which areas to address as a priority, which are not urgent, and which could be improved but also could remain unchanged. Such discussions are likely to reveal faculty beliefs and values about nursing practice, educational approaches, and student-teacher relationships, all of which provide an excellent opportunity to return to and reflect on the philosophy.

The goal of curriculum evaluation is not to make everyone happy, as that is impossible. However, if the most significant guiding principles are "What is best for student learning?" and "What will help us best prepare students for today's and tomorrow's world?" consensus can be reached and appropriate curriculum refinements or revisions can be made.

Course Report

Semester/Section:

Faculty:

Course:

Delivery method:

Number of students enrolled:

Prerequisite(s):

Corequisite(s):

Previous learning experiences prepared students to be successful in the course.

Strongly Disagree	Disagree	Agree	Strongly Agree
☐	☐	☐	☐

Comments:

Students achieved stated learning outcomes for the course.

Strongly Disagree	Disagree	Agree	Strongly Agree
☐	☐	☐	☐

Comments:

FIGURE 2.1 Example course report. (*continued*)

Course expectations and outcomes clearly aligned with level objectives.

Strongly Disagree	Disagree	Agree	Strongly Agree
☐	☐	☐	☐

Comments:

Clinical experiences (sites used, staff relationships, etc.) enhanced students' learning.

Strongly Disagree	Disagree	Agree	Strongly Agree
☐	☐	☐	☐

Comments:

Teaching strategies used in the course.

Strategy	Number of times used	Summary of student performance
Lecture		
Online forums/discussion		
Case studies		
Videos		
Internet resources		
Mobile apps		
Gaming		
Simulation		
Problem-based learning		
Other:		

Faculty Reflections on effectiveness of teaching/learning strategies used:

Assessment/Evaluation methods used in the course.

Evaluation method	Number of times used	Summary of student performance
Exam		
Quiz		
Practice questions		
Case study		
Group project		
Major writing assignment		
Minor writing assignment		
Skills assessment		
Other:		

Faculty Reflections on effectiveness of evaluation methods used:

Additional Considerations:

What new teaching/learning strategies were used? Why were they selected? How were they received by students and faculty? How effective were they?

What new assessment/evaluation strategies were used? Why were they selected? How were they received by students and faculty? How effective were they?

Were formative evaluations done during the course? What changes were made during the course in response to that feedback from students?

Summarize the feedback—positive and negative—provided by students on the end-of-term course evaluation form.

What changes are recommended for future offerings of this course?

Summarize any feedback from clinical partners, course collaborators, guest speakers, etc.

Please provide any other comments about the course that will be helpful for future planning.

FIGURE 2.1 Example course report.

Summary

In conclusion, it is important to remember that curriculum evaluation is an ongoing and complex process that must involve all faculty. Input must be sought from all stakeholders—students, faculty, clinical partners, employers, and administrators—to obtain a comprehensive view of what is effective and what needs improvement. Additionally, it is critical to keep in mind that a change in one component of the curriculum is very likely to impact other components. The curriculum should be conceptualized as a gestalt, and attention should be paid to the complex and dynamic interactions among students, teachers, learning experiences, the material to be learned, and the values to be reflected upon.

Curriculum revisions should be implemented thoughtfully, and faculty should be sensitive to avoid allowing existing practices to become "carved in stone." Instead, a curriculum should be thought of as a living, dynamic entity that evolves along with the needs of society, the nursing profession, individual schools, and changing student populations. Nursing students and the patients, families, and communities for whom they will care, deserve nothing less.

References

Accreditation Commission for Education in Nursing. (2020). *ACEN™ Accreditation manual—Section III. Standards & Criteria*. https://www.acenursing.org/acen-accreditation-manual-standards-and-criteria/

Adams, M. H., & Valiga, T. M. (2021). *Achieving distinction in nursing education*. National League for Nursing.

Commission on Collegiate Nursing Accreditation. (2018, Amended). *Standards for accreditation of baccalaureate and graduate nursing programs*. https://www.aacnnursing.org/Portals/42/CCNE/PDF/Standards-Final-2018.pdf

Coomer, M. N., Skelton, S. M., Kyser, T. S., Warren, C., & Thorius, K. A. K. (2017).

Assessing Bias in Standards & Curricular Materials Tool. https://greatlakesequity.org/resource/assessing-bias-standards-and-curricular-materials

Ironside, P. M. (2004). "Covering content" and teaching thinking: Deconstructing the additive curriculum. *Journal of Nursing Education, 43*(1), 5–12. doi: 10.3928/01484834-20040101-02

National League for Nursing (NLN). (2020). *Hallmarks of excellence in nursing education model*. http://www.nln.org/professional-development-programs/teaching-resources/hallmarks-of-excellence

National League for Nursing Commission for Nursing Education Accreditation. (2016). *Accreditation standards for nursing education programs*. https://cnea.nln.org/standards-of-accreditation

Northwestern University Feinberg School of Medicine. (2021). *Inclusive and bias free checklist*. Accessed December 30, 2021.

https://www.feinberg.northwestern.edu/md-education/learning-environment/checklist.html

Sherman, M. D., Ricco, J., Nelson, S. C., Nezhad, S. J., & Prasad, S. (2019). Implicit bias training in a residency program: Aiming for enduring effects. *Family Medicine, 51*(8), 677–681. https://doi.org/10.22454/FamMed.2019.947255

Tanner, C. A. (2004). The meaning of curriculum: Content to be covered or stories to be heard? *Journal of Nursing Education, 43*(1), 3–4. doi: 10.3928/01484834-20040101-04

Valiga, T. M. (2015). Rethinking prerequisites. *Journal of Nursing Education, 54*(4), 183–184. doi: 10.3928/01484834-20150318

Valiga, T. M. (2020). Philosophical foundations of the curriculum. In D. M. Billings & J. A. Halstead, *Teaching in nursing: A guide for faculty* (6th ed., pp. 135–146). Elsevier.

3

Formulating Evaluation and Survey Questions

Lisa D. Brodersen, EdD, PhD, RN, CNE

After establishing the purpose of the program evaluation, the next step is to formulate the *evaluation questions*. Evaluation questions are interrogative statements about the implementation and outcomes of a program (Rossi et al., 2019). In nursing education, answers to evaluation questions inform judgments about the merit, value, and overall quality of a nursing program based on established institutional goals, program outcomes, accreditation criteria, and regulatory standards (Welch, 2021). More specifically, answers to evaluation questions indicate:

> The extent to which students are learning nursing competencies, achieving program outcomes, and attaining licensure or certification.

> How well faculty have designed and implemented the curriculum and the extent to which it is preparing students for nursing practice.

> If the school of nursing has the necessary administrative, fiscal, and physical resources to support teaching and learning and the extent to which those resources are used efficiently and effectively.

Evaluation questions should not be confused with survey questions (Centers for Disease Control and Prevention [CDC], 2013; Wingate & Schroeter, 2007). Evaluation questions are broader than survey questions; however, answering evaluation questions often involves administering surveys. Surveys contain specific questions or other types of items, each of which is designed to measure a single data point (Waltz et al., 2017). Answering evaluation questions may require administering one or more surveys. Furthermore, one or more questions on a survey may be needed to answer an evaluation question. Nevertheless, good evaluation questions and good survey questions are essential to a good evaluation. The purpose of this chapter is to provide guidelines for formulating good evaluation questions *and* good survey questions.

RELATIONSHIP OF EVALUATION QUESTIONS TO OTHER COMPONENTS OF EVALUATION

Evaluation questions are ultimately determined by the purpose of the evaluation (Rossi et al., 2019). In nursing education, the purpose of program evaluation is to systematically evaluate (a) compliance with accreditation and regulatory standards, (b) the achievement of program outcomes, and (c) the performance on other indicators of program effectiveness and quality included in the program's systematic evaluation plan. Therefore, common sources of evaluation questions include a program's systematic evaluation plan and the standards of its accrediting agencies and state boards of nursing (Oermann & Gaberson, 2021). To some extent, evaluation questions are implied by these indicators and standards, in which case they may never be explicitly written. However, problems, events, or circumstances that require investigation may emerge during the day-to-day operations of the nursing program. Such occurrences may not be addressed by the systematic evaluation plan, in which case evaluation questions are needed to guide the evaluation. Table 3.1 provides examples of evaluation questions derived from accreditation standards organized by areas of accreditation.

Regardless of their sources, good evaluation questions are needed because they are the starting point for program evaluation, providing the organizing framework for the evaluation and directing decisions about the evaluation plan, including measurement, data analysis, and dissemination of findings (Rossi et al., 2019; Wilce et al., 2021). Derived from the purpose of the evaluation, evaluation questions indicate the design of the evaluation, informing the selection of the indicators of program performance, effectiveness, and quality. In turn, indicators inform the methods used to collect and analyze the data that will ultimately answer the evaluation questions. Lastly, the evaluation questions may provide the organizing scheme for disseminating the evaluation findings.

CHARACTERISTICS OF GOOD EVALUATION QUESTIONS

Good evaluation questions are "meaningful, important, feasible to answer...and likely to provide useful information to primary intended users and other stakeholders" (Fitzpatrick et al., 2011, p. 314). In other words, good evaluation questions are "evaluative" (Wingate & Schoeter, 2007). Evaluative evaluation questions lead to evidence that faculty and administrators can use to judge the strengths and weaknesses of the nursing program, thereby guiding their decisions about changes needed to improve program effectiveness and quality.

Evaluation experts have created checklists to guide formulation and refinement of good evaluation questions. The *Evaluation Questions Checklist for Program Evaluation*, developed by the Western Michigan University Evaluation Center (Wingate & Schroeter, 2007), defines five criteria for good evaluation questions: Good evaluation questions should be evaluative, pertinent, reasonable, specific, and answerable. The *Checklist for Assessing Your Evaluation Questions* was created by the Center for Disease Control and Prevention's National Asthma Control Program (CDC, 2013). This tool defines four criteria for good evaluation questions based on stakeholder engagement, appropriate fit, relevance, and feasibility. Both tools can be adapted to the specific type of program being evaluated, are available online, and require no permission to use.

TABLE 3.1

Examples of Evaluation Questions Derived from Accreditation Standards

Area of Accreditation	Standards	Examples of Evaluation Questions
Mission & Governance	ACEN 1. Mission and Administrative Capacity	Is the mission of the program congruent with the governing institution's mission, goals, and values?
		Do the program and its governing institution have enough administrative capacity to ensure effective delivery of the program and achievement of program outcomes?
	CNEA II: Culture of Integrity and Accountability–Mission, Governance, and Resources	Do the program and its governing institution share a commitment to a culture of integrity and accountability?
		Are the mission and goals of the program aligned with the mission and goals of its governing institution?
	CCNE I. Program Quality: Mission and Governance	Are the program's mission, goals, and outcomes congruent with those of the parent institution?
		Do the program's mission, goals, and outcomes reflect relevant professional standards?
		Do the program's mission, goals, and outcomes reflect the needs and expectations of its communities of interest?
Faculty	ACEN 2. Faculty and Staff	Are there enough qualified and credentialed faculty to achieve student learning and program outcomes?
		Are there enough qualified support staff?
	CNEA III. Culture of Excellence and Caring–Faculty	Is the program committed to creating a culture of excellence and caring and supportive of faculty outcomes?
	CCNE II. Program Quality: Institutional Commitment and Resources	Are there enough faculty to achieve the program's mission, goals, and outcomes?
		Are faculty academically and experientially qualified to fulfill their teaching roles?
Students	ACEN 3. Students	Do student policies and services support achievement of student learning and program outcomes?
	CNEA IV. Culture of Excellence and Caring–Students	Is the program committed to creating a caring, culturally responsive environment that fosters student success?

(continued)

TABLE 3.1

Examples of Evaluation Questions Derived from Accreditation Standards *(Continued)*

Area of Accreditation	Standards	Examples of Evaluation Questions
	CCNE I–IV	Are students involved in shared governance and program improvement?
		Do teaching practices and the teaching-learning environment foster achievement of student outcomes?
		Do students achieve the program outcomes?
Curriculum	ACEN 4. Curriculum	Does the curriculum support achievement of student learning and program outcomes?
		Is the curriculum consistent with safe practice in current healthcare settings?
	CNEA V. Culture of Learning and Diversity–Curriculum and Evaluation Processes	Do the program's curriculum and evaluation processes demonstrate a culture of learning and diversity?
	CCNE III. Program Quality: Curriculum and Teaching-Learning Practices	Does the curriculum reflect the program's mission, goals, and outcomes?
		Does the curriculum reflect professional nursing standards, guidelines, and the needs of communities of interest?
		Are teaching-learning practices appropriate to foster achievement of student outcomes?
Resources	ACEN 5. Resources	Are fiscal, physical, and learning resources sustainable and sufficient to ensure the achievement of student learning and program outcomes?
	CNEA II: Culture of Integrity and Accountability–Mission, Governance, and Resources	Do the program and its governing institution demonstrate a culture of integrity and accountability in resource allocation?
	CCNE II. Program Quality: Institutional Commitment and Resources	Does the parent institution support the nursing program with the resources needed to achieve its mission, goals, and outcomes?
		Do faculty and staff enable the program to achieve its mission, goals, and outcomes?
Outcomes	ACEN 6. Outcomes	Does program evaluation demonstrate that students achieve the end-of-program learning outcomes and competencies?
		Does the program have a current systematic plan of evaluation?

TABLE 3.1		
Examples of Evaluation Questions Derived from Accreditation Standards *(Continued)*		
Area of Accreditation	**Standards**	**Examples of Evaluation Questions**
	CNEA I. Culture of Excellence–Program Outcomes	Does the program demonstrate commitment to continuous quality improvement through ongoing, systematic assessment and evaluation of institutional and program outcomes?
	CCNE IV. Program Effectiveness: Assessment and Achievement of Program Outcomes	Is the program fulfilling its mission and goals by achieving the expected program outcomes? Is program effectiveness data used to foster program improvement?

ACEN, Accreditation Commission for Education in Nursing (2020); CCNE, Commission on Collegiate Nursing Education (2018); CNEA, National League for Nursing Commission on Collegiate Nursing Accreditation (2021).

A synthesis of expert guidance about the characteristics of good evaluation questions suggests that in addition to being clear, concise, and grammatically written, they must be *salient*, *focused*, and *productive*. Salient evaluation questions reflect the purpose of the evaluation and the priorities and interests of students, faculty, program administrators, and other stakeholders (CDC, 2013). They yield answers that are important and meaningful to stakeholders (Fitzpatrick et al., 2011). Focused evaluation questions indicate who or what will be evaluated and how it will be evaluated. They suggest the criteria that indicate if a standard or outcome was met (Rossi et al., 2019; Wingate & Schroeter, 2007). Productive evaluation questions are measurable and, therefore, answerable (Rossi et al., 2019; Wingate & Schroeter, 2007). Moreover, they yield valid and useful evidence that informs stakeholders' judgments about the quality of the program and decisions about program change (Fitzpatrick et al., 2011; Rossi et al., 2019). Productive evaluation questions are measurable because they can be operationalized with data collection methods, and sufficient human, physical, and fiscal resources are available to manage and analyze the data needed to answer them (CDC, 2013; Fitzpatrick et al., 2011; Wingate & Schroeter, 2007).

Guidelines for Formulating Good Evaluation Questions

Formulating evaluation questions should be a systematic process. It begins by working with stakeholders to determine the purpose and focus of the evaluation (Fitzpatrick et al., 2011). If the evaluation is driven by accreditation or regulatory standards, evaluation questions can be derived from the standards by converting them into one or more evaluation questions. If these evaluation questions are too broad, more specific, measurable evaluation questions can be formulated from the quality indicators that accompany the standards.

Ultimately, evaluation questions should align with the purpose of the evaluation and needs of stakeholders. The following steps facilitate the formulation of good evaluation questions (CDC, 2018):

1. Consider the purpose of the evaluation, who will use the results, and how the results will be used.
2. Identify the specific components of the project, service, or initiative to be evaluated (e.g., specific activities, processes, outcomes, intervening factors).
3. Isolate the specific attributes to be evaluated (e.g., attitudes, perceptions, opinions, achievements).
4. Formulate salient, focused, and productive evaluation questions that represent the specific attributes to be evaluated.

Identifying Appropriate Indicators

Evaluation questions are essentially inquiries about performance on a standard or outcome (Rossi et al., 2019). Sometimes evaluation questions have ambiguous terms (Wilce et al., 2021), which is why *indicators* are needed. Indicators are the criteria that signify if a standard or outcome was met. In other words, indicators represent the desired or ideal answers to the evaluation questions. Indicators are associated with expected levels of achievement, also called targets or benchmarks (Beasley et al., 2018).

If a nursing program's systematic evaluation plan is driven by accreditation and regulatory standards, the indicators for the standards in each area of accreditation will be prespecified, as shown in Table 3.2. However, faculty may need to evaluate other components of the nursing program that are not explicitly represented in the systematic evaluation plan (e.g., peer tutoring program, summer externship program). New evaluation questions will be raised, and faculty will need to identify appropriate indicators, measures, and targets to answer them, as illustrated in Table 3.3.

The same stakeholders involved in formulating the evaluation question should also be involved in identifying appropriate indicators and targets (Fitzpatrick et al., 2011; Rossi et al., 2019). The starting point for identifying indicators is the evaluation question, derived from the purpose of the evaluation. The indicators should align with the concepts in the evaluation question in measurable terms. Targets should be relevant and denote high, but realistic expectations. The following steps can be followed to identify appropriate indicators and targets:

1. Review the evaluation question to identify the specific attributes to be evaluated (e.g., attitudes, perceptions, opinions, achievements).
2. Formulate an indicator of each evaluative attribute in the question.
3. Identify relevant, realistic targets for each indicator.
4. Consider the feasibility of measuring each indicator (e.g., time, resources, ethical considerations).

TABLE 3.2

Examples of Evaluation Questions and Indicators for Selected Accreditation Standards

Standard	Evaluation Questions	Indicators
ACEN 3. Students	Do student policies and services support achievement of student learning and program outcomes?	3.8. Orientation to technology is provided, and technological support is available to students.
CNEA V. Culture of Learning and Diversity—Curriculum and Evaluation Processes	Do the program's curriculum and evaluation processes demonstrate a culture of learning and diversity?	V-G. The faculty use a variety of teaching, learning, and evaluation strategies within the curriculum.
CCNE III. Program Quality: Curriculum and Teaching-Learning Practices	Does the curriculum reflect professional nursing standards, guidelines, and the needs of communities of interest?	III-H. The curriculum includes planned clinical practice experiences that enable students to integrate new knowledge and demonstrate attainment of program outcomes, foster interprofessional collaborative practice, and are evaluated by faculty.
ACEN 5. Resources	Are fiscal, physical, and learning resources sustainable and sufficient to ensure the achievement of student learning and program outcomes?	5.2. Physical resources are sufficient to ensure the achievement of the end-of-program student learning outcomes and program outcomes, and meet the needs of the faculty, staff, and students.
CNEA II: Culture of Integrity and Accountability—Mission, Governance, and Resources	Do the program and its governing institution demonstrate a culture of integrity and accountability in resource allocation?	II-C. Communities of interest provide feedback which is used to inform program decision-making about the educational preparation of students.
CCNE IV. Program Effectiveness: Assessment and Achievement of Program Outcomes	Is the program fulfilling its mission and goals by achieving the expected program outcomes?	IV.C. Licensure pass rates demonstrate program effectiveness. IV.D. Certification pass rates demonstrate program effectiveness.

ACEN, Accreditation Commission for Education in Nursing (2020); CCNE, Commission on Collegiate Nursing Education (2018); CNEA, National League for Nursing Commission on Collegiate Nursing Accreditation (2021).

CREATING AND SELECTING HIGH-QUALITY SURVEY QUESTIONS

After formulating good evaluation questions and identifying appropriate indicators, the next step in the evaluation process is to design the evaluation. Designing the evaluation entails identifying or creating the assessment methods, or *measures* that will operationalize the indicators and provide the evidence needed to answer the evaluation questions. Adequately answering a single evaluation question may require measuring more

TABLE 3.3

Example of an Evaluation Plan for a Nurse Externship Program

Evaluation Questions	Indicators	Targets	Measures
What is the impact of the externship on participants' confidence related to CDM?	Students will report increased self-confidence related to clinical decision-making.	Post-externship scores 15 points > pre-externship score.	NASC-CDM, self-confidence scale score (post-externship score minus pre-externship score).
What is the impact of the externship on participants' anxiety related to CDM?	Students will report decreased anxiety related to clinical decision-making.	Post-externship scores 10 points < pre-externship score.	NASC-CDM, anxiety scale (pre-externship score minus post-externship score).
What is the impact of the externship on hiring new graduates?	Number of nursing program graduates hired by the hospital will increase.	≥50% of externship participants will hire on (date or date range).	Percentage of externship participants hired (number hired divided by number of participants).
		Number of nursing program graduates hired after externship greater than mean number hired during 5-year period before externship.	Compare number of nursing program graduates hired 1 year after externship to mean number hired during 5-year period before externship.

CDM, clinical decision making; NASC-CDM, Nursing Anxiety and Self-Confidence with Clinical Decision Making Scale (White, 2014).

than one indicator (Rossi et al., 2019). Furthermore, each indicator may be operationalized with more than one measure (Beasley et al., 2018).

Some indicators, such as retention, graduation, and licensure and certification examination pass rates, are relatively simple to measure. Other indicators require more complex measurement methods, such as students' perceptions of the accessibility and adequacy of academic support services and employers' perceptions of how often and how well the program's graduates perform the program outcomes. *Surveys* are often administered to collect the data needed to measure these and other indicators of program quality that answer evaluation questions.

A survey is an assessment method used often in nursing education research and program evaluation. A typical survey includes two or more interrogative or declarative statements that are intended to elicit opinions, attitudes, perceptions, and facts from the intended respondents (Fowler, 2014). Two types of surveys are used in the evaluation of nursing education programs: interviews and questionnaires (Waltz et al., 2017). The most obvious difference between interviews and questionnaires is that an interview is a verbal interaction between an interviewer and one or more respondents that may occur face-to-face, by telephone, or through a video conferencing platform, whereas a questionnaire is a paper or online form usually completed by a single respondent. Both methods have their virtues and shortcomings, but one particularly important feature they share is the need for good survey questions (Dillman et al., 2014).

STEPS FOR CREATING HIGH-QUALITY SURVEY QUESTIONS

Without good survey questions, respondents may not understand the question and may give an erroneous or biased answer, or they may skip the question altogether (Fowler, 2014). Moreover, bad survey questions are bad measures of indicators, resulting in bad answers to evaluation questions. Like writing evaluation questions, writing survey questions should be a systematic process (Waltz et al., 2017). Before writing survey questions, these preliminary steps should be taken: (1) scrutinize the indicators, (2) find existing survey questions, and (3) create high-quality survey questions.

Scrutinize the Indicators

The indicators suggest, either explicitly or implicitly, variables that could be measured to assess the indicator. For example, the National League for Nursing Commission for Nursing Education Accreditation (CNEA, 2021) Standard I quality indicator, I-F. Faculty, students, alumni, and employers express satisfaction with program effectiveness, clearly suggests measurement of satisfaction with program effectiveness in three groups of stakeholders.

Select Existing Survey Questions

Before resorting to writing survey questions to measure indicators, investigate the availability of existing surveys with questions that measure the variables in the indicators. There may be commercially available surveys that can be purchased by the nursing program (e.g., student, faculty, and employer opinion or satisfaction surveys), or it might be possible to obtain permission to borrow and adapt a survey developed by another nursing program.

Create High-Quality Survey Questions

If there is no existing survey with questions to measure the indicators, or it is not possible to purchase and/or adapt an existing survey, the alternative is to write the survey questions. Much like writing good test items, writing a survey question is a task that should not be taken lightly if the intent is to craft high-quality questions. Decisions must be made about the type of question and how respondents will be expected to answer. Furthermore, the questions must be carefully crafted to elicit valid and meaningful responses. The following sections cover the basic types of survey questions and guidelines for writing them well.

TYPES OF SURVEY QUESTIONS

Survey questions are broadly categorized as (a) open-ended or (b) closed-ended (Waltz et al., 2017). Both open- and closed-ended survey questions start with a stem, which is the part that includes the actual question along with any additional information to facilitate the respondents' understanding of what they are being asked (Dillman et al., 2014). The next sections cover the differences between open- and closed-ended questions. Box 3.1 contains examples of common survey question types.

Open-Ended Questions

Because they provide no response options, open-ended questions permit (or require) respondents to devise their own answers (Dillman et al., 2014). Open-ended questions can be written to elicit brief or detailed responses. The main reason to include an open-ended question on a survey is if too little is known about the question topic to create a list of response options or if a very detailed answer is desired. Because they include no response options, open-ended questions are somewhat easier to write than closed ended questions. However, they are not necessarily easier to answer. If respondents are

---

BOX 3.1

Types of Survey Questions

Open-Ended

What are your perceptions of the nursing program? Please comment on the strengths and challenges you experienced with individual courses, faculty, staff, and resources.

> [ ]

In what area of practice do you plan to seek employment as a registered nurse?

> [ ]

Multiple-Response

In what setting(s) are you currently employed as a nurse? Select all that apply.

- [ ] Acute Care (e.g., inpatient, hospital)
- [ ] Ambulatory Care (e.g., community or home health)
- [ ] Education (e.g., school of nursing)
- [ ] Long Term Care (e.g., skilled nursing, rehab, nursing home)
- [ ] Other (please specify)

  > [ ]

Nominal Response

What are your plans regarding future education?

- ◯ Immediately pursue a nursing graduate degree
- ◯ Pursue a nursing graduate degree within 5 years
- ◯ Pursue a non-health related graduate degree
- ◯ Do not intend to pursue a graduate degree

BOX 3.1

Types of Survey Questions *(Continued)*

Ordinal-Response, Numeric

Slider

How likely are you to recommend this nursing program to a friend or family member who is interested in nursing? Move the slider to choose your response.

0 (not at all likely)　　　　　　　　　　　　　　　　10 (extremely likely)

5-point numeric response scale

How well did the BSN program prepare you to use evidence-based practice in nursing care?

◯ 1 (Not well at all)　◯ 2　◯ 3　◯ 4　◯ 5 (Extremely well)

Traditional 100 mm Visual Analog Scale (VAS)

How much anxiety did you experience *during* the objective structured clinical exam? Draw a slash through the horizontal line to rate your anxiety.

No Anxiety |　　　　　　　　　　　　　　　　　　　　　| Extreme Anxiety

Ordinal-Response, Likert

Bipolar response options (weak/strong; agree/disagree)

How much did your educational experience at this college influence your desire to provide service to your community?

◯ Very strong influence

◯ Strong influence

◯ Moderate influence

◯ Weak influence

◯ No influence

Assuming some additional preparation and study, do you agree or disagree that your education has prepared you to succeed on the licensure exam?

Strongly agree	Agree	Neither agree nor disagree	Disagree	Strongly disagree
◯	◯	◯	◯	◯

Filter

Are you currently employed as a nurse?

◯ Yes ──────────────────→

◯ No

│
↓

If you are not currently employed in nursing, are you looking for employment in nursing?

◯ Yes

◯ No

What is your primary nursing practice setting?

◯ Acute Care (e.g., inpatient, hospital)

◯ Ambulatory Care (e.g., community or home health)

◯ Education (e.g., school of nursing)

◯ Long Term Care (e.g., skilled nursing, rehab, nursing home)

◯ Other (please specify)

[   ]

(continued)

BOX 3.1

Types of Survey Questions *(Continued)*

Ranking

Of the following hospital clinical areas you experienced during the nursing program, which did you prefer most? Rank the areas in order of your preference (1 = most preferred, 7 = least preferred).

Critical care

Emergency

Med-surg

Maternal-newborn

Mental health

PACU

Pediatrics

Of the following hospital clinical areas you experienced during the nursing program, which 3 areas did you prefer most? Rank the top 3 areas in order of your preference (1 = most preferred, 3 = third most preferred).

Critical care

Emergency

Med-surg

Maternal-newborn

Mental health

PACU

Pediatrics

Matrix

Do you agree or disagree with the following statements about this college?

	Strongly agree	Agree	Disagree	Strongly disagree	Not applicable/do not know
The Financial Aid Office has been helpful with financial needs.	○	○	○	○	○
The Registrar's Office, including the academic registration centers (ARC), has been helpful with registration needs.	○	○	○	○	○
The library staff has been helpful with library and resource needs.	○	○	○	○	○
The facilities (buildings, classrooms, library, etc.) have met my needs.	○	○	○	○	○

Questions adapted from Allen College-UnityPoint Health, Waterloo, IA, surveys with permission. Reprinted by permission of Allen College-UnityPoint Health, February 28, 2022.

not provided a fixed list of response options, they may provide too much information, or they may not be motivated to put the necessary effort into their response, give an incomplete or sketchy answer, or skip the question altogether.

Open-ended questions can also be cumbersome to answer on handheld electronic devices (e.g., smartphone, tablet). In addition to not necessarily being easy to answer, the responses to some open-ended questions can be difficult to analyze and aggregate, particularly when they are varied and/or lengthy. Despite their drawbacks, it can be useful to include open-ended questions on a survey to elicit information about a topic when too little is known about it to create response options. Open-ended questions also permit respondents to explain their response to closed-ended questions or to offer additional information that may not have been addressed by other questions on the survey.

Closed-Ended Questions

Closed-ended questions are also called *forced-choice* or *fixed-alternative* questions (Waltz et al., 2017). In addition to the stem, closed-ended questions include two or more response options. Although considered more difficult to write than open-ended questions, analysis and aggregation of responses are considerably less time-consuming, especially when the survey is administered using an online survey platform (e.g., SurveyMonkey®, Qualtrics®).

High-quality closed-ended questions can be challenging to write; not only must the stem be clearly written, but the response options must be *collectively exhaustive* as well as *mutually exclusive*. A collectively exhaustive list of response options includes all plausible answers to the question. Box 3.2 provides examples of closed-ended questions that are not mutually exclusive or collectively exhaustive.

Because it can be difficult to compile a set of response options that are collectively exhaustive, a common strategy is to include other-please specify, don't know, or undecided as response options, which gives respondents an answer option when none of the other options apply (Dillman et al., 2014). However, don't know and undecided should be included as a response option only if they are plausible, that is, if some respondents truly might not know or truly have not decided (Patten, M. L. 2014). If it is appropriate to include other-please specify, don't know, or undecided as response options, they should be included at the end of the list of options (Dillman et al., 2014).

Mutually exclusive response options are unique and distinct from one another, meaning there is no redundancy or overlap between options. Closed-ended questions can be broadly categorized as *multiple-choice* or *ranking questions*. Types of multiple-choice questions include *nominal response*, *ordinal response*, *numeric rating*, and *Likert* questions. Furthermore, multiple-choice questions may be presented in a *matrix*. Multiple-choice and ranking question types are described in the next sections.

Multiple-Choice Questions

Multiple-choice questions are closed-ended questions that can be classified as *single-response* or *multiple-response* questions. With single-response questions, respondents are asked to select only one answer, whereas multiple-response questions may permit

BOX 3.2

Survey Question Problems and Solutions

Survey Question	Problems	Solution
Approximately how many hours of community service have you done in the past 12 months? ○ 0 hours ○ 1–5 hours ○ 5–10 hours ○ 10–15 hours ○ 15–20 hours	The response options overlap: they are not mutually exclusive. There is no option for respondents who have done more than 20 hours of community service; response options are not collectively exhaustive.	Approximately how many hours of community service have you done in the past 12 months? ○ 0 hours ○ 1–4 hours ○ 5–9 hours ○ 10–14 hours ○ 15–19 hours ○ 20 or more hours
Considering the excellent education you received in this nursing program, how likely are you to recommend it to a friend or family member? ○ Very likely ○ Likely ○ Neither likely nor unlikely ○ Unlikely ○ Very unlikely	The question stem is not worded neutrally (i.e., it is biased) and could imply that respondents should choose one of the more favorable responses; it is a leading question. The question stem is also less specific than it should be. It does not provide the context for recommending the program (e.g., interest in nursing). The response options include a neutral option, but it does not seem plausible that the respondent would not be either likely or unlikely to recommend the program to a family member or friend.	Considering your experience in the nursing program, how likely or unlikely are you to recommend it to a friend or family member who is interested in nursing? ○ Very likely ○ Likely ○ Unlikely ○ Very unlikely
If you were aware that one of your classmates had cheated on an exam, would you report the cheater to faculty? ○ Yes ○ No	The wording of this question stem implies judgment. The response options are not collectively exhaustive. It is possible the respondent may be ambivalent or unsure of what action they would take.	If a nursing student is aware of a classmate cheating on an exam, do you agree or disagree that the nursing student should report the classmate to faculty? ○ Strongly agree ○ Agree ○ Disagree ○ Strongly disagree ○ Undecided

BOX 3.2

Survey Question Problems and Solutions *(Continued)*

Survey Question	Problems	Solution
Do you disagree that the instructor did not use a variety of teaching strategies? ○ Strongly agree ○ Agree ○ Neither agree nor disagree ○ Disagree ○ Strongly disagree	The question stem is not worded neutrally, nor is it balanced with the response options. The question stem lacks context; making it somewhat vague regarding when a variety of teaching strategies may have been used. The response options include a neutral option, but it does not seem plausible that the respondent would not agree or disagree regarding the variety of teaching strategies.	Thinking back on the semester, do you agree or disagree that the instructor used a variety of teaching strategies? ○ Strongly agree ○ Agree ○ Disagree ○ Strongly disagree
About how often during the semester do you visit the college library and use the computers in the college computer lab? ○ Daily ○ A few times a week ○ About once a week ○ A few times a month ○ Once a month ○ Less than once a month ○ Never	This question stem contains two questions. Separate questions should be asked about the frequency with which the two campus resources are used.	About how often during the semester do you visit the college library? ○ Daily ○ A few times a week ○ About once a week ○ A few times a month ○ Once a month ○ Less than once a month ○ Never About how often during the semester do you use the computers in the college computer lab? ○ Daily ○ A few times a week ○ About once a week ○ A few times a month ○ Once a month ○ Less than once a month ○ Never

(continued)

BOX 3.2

Survey Question Problems and Solutions *(Continued)*

Survey Question	Problems	Solution
As an employer of a graduate of the DNP program, are you satisfied with the collaboration outcome? ○ Always ○ Usually ○ Sometimes ○ Rarely ○ Never	The question stem is concise and brief but vague. The respondent may not be familiar with the DNP program's collaboration outcome. The relevance of the collaboration outcome to the DNP graduate is not explicit. The response options are not consistent with the question stem.	As an employer of a DNP program graduate, how satisfied or dissatisfied are you with the graduate's collaboration within interprofessional teams to manage and improve health care services for individuals, families and populations? ○ Very satisfied ○ Satisfied ○ Dissatisfied ○ Very dissatisfied

DNP, doctor of nursing practice.
Questions adapted from Allen College-UnityPoint Health, Waterloo, IA, surveys with permission. Reprinted by permission of Allen College-UnityPoint Health, February 28, 2022.

respondents to select all that apply or restrict them to a specified number of answers. In paper-based and online surveys, the response options for single-response questions are typically accompanied by a circle or radio button to indicate where respondents would mark or click to select their response. In contrast, the response options for multiple-response questions are usually accompanied by square checkboxes. Single-response multiple-choice questions can be further classified as *nominal* or *ordinal* response questions. Box 3.1 provides examples of nominal and ordinal single-response multiple-choice questions.

Multiple-response questions are often used to combine several survey questions that require a dichotomous response (yes/no, true/false, agree/disagree) into a single question. However, respondents may not answer this type of multiple-response question as accurately as they would a series of yes/no questions because there may be a tendency for respondents to choose options near the top of the list while disregarding options lower in the list (Dillman et al., 2014; Pew Research Center, 2019). Asking a series of yes/no questions may be a wiser strategy because respondents might be more likely to consider and answer each question. If multiple-response questions are used in a paper-based survey, the question stem and response options should cover no more than one-half page. Questions spanning more than one-half page should be divided into two or more shorter multiple-response questions or converted to single-response, yes/no questions. If using an online survey platform, the response options in a multiple-response question can be ordered randomly to control the tendency to disregard response options lower in the list. Box 3.1 includes an example of a multiple-response question.

Nominal Response Questions

Nominal response questions offer response options that have no intrinsic sequence or order (Dillman et al., 2014). In other words, there is no natural hierarchy for the response options. For example, if graduating students were asked on an exit survey, In what practice setting do you plan to work?, the response options (e.g., medical clinic, community health, hospital, long-term care, etc.) would not represent categories that have any meaningful order, other than alphabetical. Nominal response questions can be either single-response, multiple-response, or ranking questions (Dillman et al., 2014). Box 3.1 includes examples of nominal single-response questions.

Ordinal Response Questions

Ordinal response questions, also called rating scales, are a type of single-response, multiple-choice question used to measure the amount or intensity of subjective variables, such as attitudes, opinions, concerns, emotions, sensations, behaviors, and attributes. The response options in ordinal questions have an intrinsic sequence or order (Dillman et al., 2014). Numeric rating questions and Likert questions are types of ordinal response questions. Ordinal questions may measure *unipolar* or *bipolar* dimensions of a variable. Unipolar questions measure one dimension of a variable on a continuum anchored by its minimum and maximum extremes (e.g., *not at all likely* to *extremely likely*). In contrast, bipolar scales represent the continuums of two opposite dimensions of a variable and are anchored by the maximum extremes of each dimension (e.g., *extremely difficult* to *extremely easy; strongly agree* to *strongly disagree*). Box 3.1 includes examples of ordinal single-response questions.

Numeric rating questions are single-choice, unipolar, ordinal questions that quantify the amount or intensity of attitudes, opinions, physical sensations, and emotions. To answer the question, respondents select a number from a given range of numeric response options. The lowest and highest response options are defined to give the respondent some guidance on the meaning of the number they select. The range of response options on numeric rating questions typically varies from 5 to 10 but may be 100 or more. For example, on an end-of-program exit survey, graduating students might be asked to use a 7-point scale of 1 (not important) to 7 (extremely important) to rate the importance of various aspects of the curriculum to their academic success. This scale could also be reduced to five options or expanded to 10 or more. Box 3.1 provides examples of numeric rating questions, including the visual analog scale (VAS).

A VAS is a type of numeric rating scale on which the response options traditionally range from 0 to 100 (Dillman et al., 2014). The VAS is typically used in research to measure physical sensations or emotions (Waltz et al., 2017). Respondents rate the level of intensity of the specified sensation or emotion by marking a 100-mm horizontal line somewhere between the anchors of 0 and 100. In a paper-based survey, the evaluator measures the distance from the 0 point to the mark to determine the score. For example, if the measured distance from the 0 point to the respondent's mark was 79 mm, the score for the variable would be 79. Online survey platforms offer the VAS as a "slider" question, which requires the respondent to move the slider to a point on the horizontal continuum that represents their rating (Box 3.1). An advantage of the slider question in online surveys is that it automatically calculates the score. A disadvantage of slider questions is that they may be difficult for respondents to complete on a smartphone or tablet.

Likert Questions

Likert questions are named after Renis Likert, a social psychologist whose work in the 1930s on the psychometric properties of attitude scales (Likert, R. 1932) evolved into what is known as Likert or Likert-type questions today. Likert questions are crafted to assess the bipolar or unipolar dimensions of a variety of attitudes (e.g., agreement, approval, satisfaction, frequency, difficulty, importance, quality, etc.). Like numeric rating questions, the response options for Likert questions are associated with a number or score (e.g., strongly disagree = 1, strongly agree = 5). However, the response options are presented as words, so when respondents rate the intensity or amount of the attitude of interest, they base their rating on the meaning of the words, rather than a number.

Likert questions may have as few as four response options, but experts advise four to five for a unipolar question and five to seven for a bipolar question (Dillman et al., 2014). Bipolar Likert questions with five or seven response options have a neutral point, usually denoted as neutral or neither/nor (i.e., neither agree nor disagree). Like don't know response options, neutral response options should be included only if it is plausible that some respondents may truly be neutral or undecided (Patten, 2014). Unlike don't know response options, neutral response options should be sequenced at the midpoint, not the end of the set of response options (Dillman et al., 2014).

Matrix Questions

Two or more multiple-choice questions with the same set of response options can be combined in a *matrix* under a single question stem. The stem poses a general question to be answered for each topic (e.g., How satisfied or dissatisfied are you with the following aspects of the course?). The topics are presented as brief phrases listed in the first column of the matrix under the stem. The response options comprise the column headings (e.g., very satisfied, satisfied, neither satisfied nor dissatisfied, dissatisfied, very dissatisfied). Like multiple-response questions, matrix questions have some drawbacks (Dillman et al., 2014). For example, there might be a tendency for respondents to choose the same response for all items or to choose a response from the wrong row (e.g., above or below the item they are answering). Another drawback is that in an online survey, a matrix question can be difficult to view fully and complete on a handheld electronic device. Survey experts advise limiting the number of items and response options in matrix questions to five or six to minimize complexity and completion time and maximize completion rate (Dillman et al., 2014; Grady, n.d.).

Ranking Questions

Ranking questions require respondents to order a set of statements according to some criterion, such as importance, magnitude, preference, or priority. Fundamentally, ranking involves placing items in a specified order. The most basic ranking method involves numbering the list of items in the desired order. Ranking questions can be difficult and time consuming for respondents to complete, resulting in incorrect or incomplete rankings (Dillman et al., 2014). There are various strategies to make ranking questions easier to complete. For example, in online surveys, respondents may be able to physically move or rearrange the items in the desired order (e.g., drag and drop). The online format also makes it possible to randomize the list of items to control the possible influence of item order on rankings. To maximize the completion and accuracy of ranking questions, the number of items should be limited (e.g., six or less). If a long list of items cannot be avoided, consider requesting that respondents rank a small number of their top preferences (e.g., three to four). Despite how ranking questions are modified to make them easier and more appealing for respondents to complete, they may be difficult to complete on handheld electronic devices (Dillman et al., 2014).

Guidelines for Creating High-Quality Survey Questions

Regardless of the survey question type, making sure they are high-quality questions is essential. Survey questions must be carefully crafted to ensure respondents understand the question, to make sure they are not being asked questions they cannot or should not answer, and to make sure they answer questions they can and should answer. Based on the recommendations of survey experts (e.g., Dillman et al., 2014; Fowler, 2014; Patten, 2014), faculty should strive to formulate survey questions that are *clear, concise, neutral*, and *necessary*.

Characteristics of Clear and Concise Survey Questions

Clear and concise survey questions begin with a grammatical stem. Although survey stems are sometimes written imperatively (i.e., as a command), survey experts specify that the stem should be written interrogatively and imperatives should be avoided (Dillman et al., 2014). Sentences should be complete but brief, consisting of words that are understood by the intended respondents. The simplest forms of terms should be used (e.g., use instead of utilize, about instead of regarding), and words with concrete meanings should be used instead of jargon, slang, or metaphorical terms. Abbreviations and acronyms should be avoided. Depending on the intended respondents, it may be wise to assess the grade-level readability or reading ease of the survey questions using an online readability checker (e.g., Flesch-Kinkaid, Fry Graph, Simple Measure of Gobbledygook Index). Flesch-Kincaid readability tools are available in Word for Microsoft word-processing software.

Each interrogative stem should include only one question. Questions that consist of two or more questions are referred to as double-barreled because they pose more than one question but permit only one answer. For example, suppose a course evaluation included the question, Do you agree or disagree that the required textbooks provide current and relevant content? (strongly agree, agree, disagree, strongly disagree). This question is asking about the currency and relevance of the textbooks' content, which are two different concepts. Furthermore, "textbooks" are plural, so if there is more than one textbook in a course, students may not have the same perception of agreement for all course textbooks. To avoid ambiguity, separate questions should be posed to assess the currency and relevance of each course textbook.

In addition to avoiding double-barreled questions, questions with double negatives or negative wording should be avoided. For example, asking, How often was the professor unavailable when needed? or Do you agree or disagree that the professor did not use a variety of teaching strategies? could be confusing to respondents, resulting in inaccurate responses. Clearer and more concise stems would be: How often was the professor available when needed and do you agree or disagree that the professor used a variety of teaching strategies?

In addition to avoiding negative wording and double negatives, the attribute in the question stem should be consistent with the attribute in the response options. For example, if respondents are being asked to indicate their satisfaction with the course textbook, the response options should consist of a satisfaction scale, not an agreement scale.

Characteristics of Neutral and Necessary Survey Questions

Not to be confused with the neutral point in a set of bipolar response options, neutral survey questions are phrased in a way that does not imply a correct or more favorable response. Neutral survey questions minimize social desirability response bias, which occurs when respondents choose a response option because they think it would convey a favorable or positive perception of themselves (Dillman et al., 2014). For example, if an alumnus reported reading three or more professional publications each month since graduating, but the true frequency is none, then the response is biased. The risk of social desirability response bias is greater for interviews than anonymous questionnaires when respondents are interacting with the questionnaire, not the interviewer (Fowler, 2014). Neutral questions also avoid implying a correct answer. For example, Do you agree the student demonstrated professionalism while on the clinical unit? could subtly imply that strongly agree or agree should be selected. To avoid leading respondents to an answer, the question could be reworded as: Do you agree or disagree the student demonstrated professionalism while on the clinical unit?

Regardless of how clear, concise, and neutral survey questions are written, they should be necessary. Necessary survey questions are those that measure the indicators that answer the evaluation questions. Questions that are merely interesting but not clearly relevant to the indicators are not needed, consume respondents' time, and should not be included in the survey. That said, survey questions that are necessary may not be relevant for every respondent. In other words, some survey questions may be relevant to some respondents, but not to others. *Filter* questions should be used to permit respondents to skip over the questions that are unnecessary for them. Filter questions, also called screening or branching questions, are used to distinguish respondents who are supposed to answer a question from those who are not.

In paper-based surveys, filter questions prompt the respondent to continue to the next question or to skip ahead to a different question. In online survey platforms (e.g., SurveyMonkey®, Qualtrics®), skip logic can be applied to a filter question. With skip logic, if a respondent's answer to a filter question disqualifies them from answering the next question, they will automatically be skipped past the next question to a question they are eligible to answer. Questions intended for some respondents, but not others are called contingency questions because answering them is contingent on the respondent's answer to a filter question. For example, asking students if they served in a leadership position while participating in service activities makes no sense if the student did not participate in any service activities while enrolled in the nursing program.

Beyond High-Quality Survey Questions: Next Steps

Creating a survey to measure indicators of program quality only starts with the formulation of survey questions. Additional steps should be taken before the survey is ready to present to the intended respondents. After determining the survey format (e.g., questionnaire or interview), the survey questions should be arranged in a sequence that will maximize the chances that respondents will complete it. For guidance about the order and sequencing of survey items, refer to Dillman et al. (2014), Fowler (2014), or Patten M. L. (2014). The survey questions should be reviewed, and the overall design and function of the survey should be tested by stakeholders, including representatives of the intended survey respondents.

Summary

Evaluation questions are broad questions about the effectiveness and quality of a nursing program. They drive the selection of indicators, which represent the desired answers to the evaluation questions. Furthermore, indicators inform the choice of evaluation methods, which often include administering surveys. High-quality survey questions are essential to a successful survey. Although evaluation questions and survey questions are distinctly different types of questions, formulating them should be a systematic process informed by established guidelines to ensure that faculty obtain the answers they need to make accurate judgments about the quality and effectiveness of the nursing program.

References

Accreditation Commission for Education in Nursing. (2020). *Accreditation manual section III: Standards and criteria.* https://www.acenursing.org/acen-accreditation-manual-standards-and-criteria/

Beasley, S. F., Farmer, S., Ard, N., & Nunn-Ellison, K. (2018). Systematic plan of evaluation part I: Assessment of end-of-program student learning outcomes. *Teaching and Learning in Nursing, 13*(1), 3–8. https://doi-org.ezp.slu.edu/10.1016/j.teln.2017.09.003

Centers for Disease Control and Prevention. (2018). *CDC Program Evaluation Framework Checklist for Step 3: Focus the Evaluation.* Retrieved January 22, 2022, from https://www.cdc.gov/eval/steps/step3/index.htm

Centers for Disease Control and Prevention, National Asthma Control Center. (2013). *Good evaluation questions: A checklist to help focus your evaluation.* Retrieved January 15, 2022, from https://www.cdc.gov/asthma/program_eval/assessingevaluation-questionchecklist.pdf

Commission on Collegiate Nursing Education. (2018). *Standards for accreditation of baccalaureate and graduate nursing programs.* https://www.aacnnursing.org/CCNE-Accreditation/Accreditation-Resources/Standards-Procedures-Guidelines

Dillman, D., Smyth, J. D., & Melani Christian, L. (2014). *Internet, phone, mail, and mixed-mode surveys: The tailored design method* (4th ed.). John Wiley & Sons.

Fitzpatrick, J. L., Sanders, J. R., & Worthen, B. R. (2011). *Program evaluation: Alternative approaches and practical guidelines* (4th ed.). Pearson.

Fowler, F. J. (2014). *Survey research methods* (5th ed.). Sage.

Grady, B. (n.d.). *What's the best way to design a matrix question?* SurveyMonkey. Retrieved January 25, 2022, from https://www.survey-monkey.com/curiosity/whats-best-way-design-matrix-question/

Likert, R. (1932). A technique for the measurement of attitudes. *Archives of Psychology*, *22*(140), 5–55.

National League for Nursing Commission for Nursing Education Accreditation. (2021). *Accreditation standards for nursing education programs*. https://cnea.nln.org/standards-of-accreditation

Oermann, M. H., & Gaberson, K. B. (2021). *Evaluation and testing in nursing education* (6th ed.). Springer Publishing Company.

Patten, M. L. (2014). *Questionnaire research: A practical guide* (4th ed.). Pyrczak Publishing.

Pew Research Center. (2019). *When online survey respondents only 'select some that apply': Forced-choice questions yield more accurate data than select-all-that-apply lists*. Retrieved February 12, 2022, from https://www.pewresearch.org/methods/2019/05/09/when-online-survey-respondents-only-select-some-that-apply/

Rossi, P. H., Lipsey, M. W., & Henry, G. T. (2019). *Evaluation: A systematic approach* (8th ed.). Sage.

Waltz, C. F., Strickland, O. L., & Lenz, E. R. (2017). *Measurement in nursing and health research* (5th ed.). Springer Publishing, LLC.

Welch, S. (2021). Program evaluation: A concept analysis. *Teaching & Learning in Nursing*, *16*(1), 81–84. https://doi.org/10.1016/j.teln.2020.08.001

White, K. A. (2014). Development and validation of a tool to measure self-confidence and anxiety in nursing students during clinical decision making. *Journal of Nursing Education*, *53*(1), 14–22. https://doi.org/10.3928/01484834-20131118-05

Wilce, M., Fierro, L. A., Gill, S., Perkins, A., Kuwahara, R., Barrera-Disler, S., Orians, C., Codd, H., Castleman, A. M., Nurmagambetov, T., & Anand, M. (2021). *Planting the seeds for high-quality program evaluation in public health*. Retrieved January 21, 2022, from https://www.cdc.gov/asthma/program_eval/planting-seeds-evaluation.htm

Wingate, L., & Schroeter, D. (2007). *Evaluation questions checklist for program evaluation*. Retrieved January 15, 2022, from http://wmich.edu/evaluation/checklists

4

Ensuring Quality of Evaluation Data

Marilyn H. Oermann, PhD, RN, FAAN, ANEF

Nurse educators need to carefully consider the methods used for collecting data for a program evaluation. Faculty, administrators, and others involved in the evaluation rely on systematically collected quality data to make good decisions about the program. This chapter provides an overview of data and data sources frequently used in program evaluation, internal and external factors that impact data quality, types of data collection methods (both quantitative and qualitative), existing tools that are available for program evaluation, and capturing data from stakeholders.

DATA AND DATA SOURCES

When planning for data collection, faculty make many decisions. They need to consider the questions to be answered and purpose of the assessment, and gather meaningful information. The type of program (e.g., prelicensure, second degree, advanced practice nursing, doctor of nursing practice [DNP]) and the reason for collecting the data (e.g., for formative evaluation during program development or to provide data for accreditation) are important considerations. Often data collection decisions are influenced by regulations and guidelines from external bodies, such as nursing accreditation agencies or state boards of nursing. The parent institution may require specific information from the nursing program, thus impacting decisions about data collection. The unique needs of the program, students, and faculty also influence decisions about data collection and selection of data sources. Lastly, fiscal, personal, and material resources and available support play an important role in decision-making about data collection. Faculty may have many ideas about possible data collection approaches, but if resources are not available to support the proposed method, alternative approaches may need to be considered. All of these factors influence the decision-making about data collection for program evaluation and can ultimately influence the quality of the data.

Because program decisions are based on the data collected, faculty need to ensure that the data provide an accurate and unbiased representation of the program, students, faculty, and other areas related to the evaluation. A variety of data sources are typically used by nursing programs as part of their program evaluation plan (Lewallen, 2015). Many schools select multiple qualitative and quantitative data collection methods

---

BOX 4.1

Sources of Data for Program Evaluation in Nursing

ePortfolios
End-of-course evaluations
Examinations (faculty made or standardized)
Focus groups
Institutional records and reports
Interviews
Nationally gathered records and reports such as National Council of State Boards of Nursing reports or
    the National Survey of Student Engagement
Projects, papers, assignments
Structured observation
Surveys

---

to ensure that they capture the information they need to make sound program decisions. Box 4.1 provides a list of some common data sources used for program evaluation in nursing.

Because of the importance of the data for decision-making, nursing programs should gather input from various perspectives while also addressing key evaluation questions and purposes. Data can be collected from a variety of stakeholders including students, faculty, administrators, clinical nurse educators, alumni, clinical partners, and employers, among others, to ensure comprehensive data and views of individuals and groups affected by the program (Box 4.2).

PSYCHOMETRIC CONSIDERATIONS

Psychometric considerations are important when making decisions about data collection for program evaluation. Individuals and groups that rely on the data for their decisions need to be confident in the findings.

BOX 4.2

Providers of Data for Program Evaluation in Nursing

Administrators
Advisory groups
Agencies (state boards of nursing, nursing accreditation bodies)
Alumni
Clinical agency (staff, preceptors, supervisors, and employers)
Faculty (clinical nurse educators, adjunct faculty, part-time faculty, educators in other roles)
Institution (in which the nursing program is housed)
Students

Reliability

One important psychometric consideration involves ensuring reliability. Reliability is the extent to which a data source yields consistent results (Stewart et al., 2021). If a survey provides reliable ratings, the ratings would be about the same if the survey was given at another time with that same group or with a similar group. A reliability coefficient of 1.00 represents perfect consistency; however, this value is rarely obtained in real educational settings. For example, standardized achievement tests used for data in a program evaluation usually have reliability coefficients in the range of 0.85 to 0.95 (Brookhart & Nitko, 2019). When faculty develop their own tests for evaluation, this same level of consistency would be unlikely because many factors can influence the scores such as intervening learning by students, differences in how the content was taught and emphasized in courses, variations in test items, and other factors.

Four types of reliability are commonly reported and include stability, equivalence, internal consistency, and interrater reliability. Stability usually involves a test-retest with correlations of those scores (Oermann & Gaberson, 2021). Another type of reliability is equivalence, but this measure requires the availability of a parallel form of an assessment. The most commonly used statistic to measure internal consistency, the third type of reliability, is Cronbach's alpha (McNeish, 2018). Although a wide range of descriptors have been used by authors to interpret acceptable, sufficient, or satisfactory reliability, a Cronbach's alpha value of 0.70 or higher is often used as a cutoff for an acceptable value (Taber, 2018). The last type of reliability that may be important to consider, particularly for open-ended assessments, is interrater reliability. If two or more raters are evaluating an item, consistency is established when there is agreement in their ratings.

Educators should be aware of factors that can influence the reliability of the results such as the length of the test or instrument (generally, the greater the number of items or questions, the greater the score reliability), similarity of the items, variability of the students, and sample size. Additionally, if items are poorly constructed or hard to understand, these can have an impact on reliability.

Validity

Another important psychometric consideration involves validity. This refers to the extent to which an instrument or test measures what it is designed for. Do the scores from the instrument or test reflect the construct being measured? For example, when interpreting results from an instrument that measures clinical judgment, do the results accurately identify skills used in clinical judgment and not some related concept such as critical thinking? Validity applies to the program evaluation design, methods, and data collection (Stewart et al., 2021).

Similar to reliability, a number of factors can impact validity, such as the content assessed and structure of the assessment. For some topics, particularly sensitive issues, participants may want to provide a socially desirable response, which may not be valid. Nurse educators can try to limit this type of response and minimize the threat to validity by ensuring confidentiality and anonymity of responses (Saleh & Bista, 2017).

Sample size also can affect validity; therefore, faculty conducting program evaluations should use as large a representative sample as possible. Ensuring that questions are complete and provide sufficient and appropriate response options also will help to ensure validity.

OTHER FACTORS THAT IMPACT DATA QUALITY

There are a variety of other factors that impact data collection and may ultimately influence the quality and quantity of data collected. Some of these factors are internal issues and are directly related to the students, faculty, and program. Others are factors that are external to the program and are related to data collected from outside of the institution.

Internal Factors

A variety of internal factors, such as the students, faculty, and program resources, may have an impact on the data collection and ultimately the quality of the data. Demographics of the students in the program may influence decisions made about data collection strategies. Student enrollment status (part- versus full-time), external demands on student time (work, family), type of program (prelicensure, second degree, advanced practice, doctoral), skill set (technology access and use), and motivation may influence the data collection methods selected for the evaluation plan. These factors also may affect student willingness to complete surveys and participate in focus groups and interviews. Are students motivated to assist faculty and invest the time to participate in the evaluation activities, particularly if they occur outside of course meeting times?

Another factor that may impact willingness to participate involves the protection of participants' identity and responses. Faculty should assess if students are comfortable providing information to them or if neutral parties should be used for data collection. Faculty need to protect the rights of students during data collection and analysis. Strategies to safeguard students include removing identifying information from data, protecting sensitive information, and assuring confidentiality. Data collection tools should be created to limit response bias, decrease the social desirability of responses, and prevent random or careless responses. Providing an appropriate environment free of distractions is also helpful in lessening the impact of internal factors. Lastly, evaluators should be sensitive to survey length and timing of administration as participants may not pay attention during or complete lengthy surveys. Survey fatigue is the phenomenon in which respondents become tired or disinterested during a survey and provide less thoughtful answers to questions, particularly in the later parts of a survey, or skip questions and leave text responses blank (Le et al., 2021). These types of responses affect the validity of the findings.

Faculty expertise and commitment to program evaluation also influence data collection. An important consideration is whether the faculty have the knowledge and skills to complete both qualitative and quantitative data collection and analysis. Do they have the technological skills to construct electronic surveys, create databases, and analyze data with spreadsheets or statistical programs? If not, are there campus resources or support services that can assist? Can workshops and training be provided to help faculty develop the skill set needed for data collection and analysis and for program evaluation? In some schools of nursing, administrators, designated individual faculty members or an evaluation committee, or a program evaluator oversee program evaluation and accreditation activities as part of their workload, while in other schools, all faculty participate in assessment and evaluation activities. Regardless of the approach used, those planning, implementing, and evaluating programs need to have the necessary knowledge and skill set to carry out these activities.

Another internal factor that may impact data quality involves resources. Does the institution have the financial resources to purchase standardized surveys, or is data collection reliant on faculty-developed materials? Is there staff support available to assist with clerical activities, such as transcription of interviews and data entry? Are resources available to conduct the best type of data collection and analysis? Internal factors are important considerations for program evaluation.

External Factors

Participants external to the institution, such as employers, preceptors, and advisory group members, can provide important perspectives about the program, students, graduates, and directions for the future. Administrators might collect information from the school's advisory group, or faculty members might interview preceptors and employers of graduates of the program. Often surveys of stakeholders external to the school are used to obtain data for program evaluation, but these typically have low response rates.

Timing of the data collection is another important external factor to consider. Faculty should ensure that those asked to complete evaluation materials have adequate time for the assessment and experience to evaluate the topic of inquiry. It also is important to avoid data collection near holidays and other busy times. Administrators and faculty responsible for program evaluation should consider these internal and external factors to help ensure the quality and quantity of data obtained.

TYPES OF DATA COLLECTION METHODS

Schools of nursing should use a variety of data collection approaches to gathering comprehensive information for program evaluation. When making decisions about data collection, faculty should consider what data are already accessible and available in the school. Using available institutional information may save cost and time, but faculty should review the data to ensure that it meets program evaluation needs. If existing instruments for collecting data are not available, faculty may need to consider adapting an instrument or developing a new one. However, creating and validating a new instrument can be challenging, particularly if faculty and others in the school lack experience in instrument development and resources are not available to guide this process. If a new instrument needs to be developed, or an existing tool is modified, the faculty should ensure it is appropriate for answering the evaluation questions and should follow established steps for developing and validating a new instrument. Kalkbrenner (2021) developed the MEASURE Approach to instrument development, which identifies seven steps for this process (Box 4.3).

BOX 4.3

Steps in Instrument Development

1. Identify the purpose and rationale for developing a new instrument or modifying an existing one (review the literature and similar instruments to confirm existing tools do not measure construct and topic of interest).
2. Identify an empirical framework (select a theory and/or synthesize findings from the literature as a framework for item development).
3. Create a theoretical blueprint (identify content and domain areas and the proportion of items for each).
4. Synthesize content and scale development (develop items and additional ones since items are typically deleted during the next step of expert review; identify types of scales).
5. Use expert reviewers (have experts review draft versions of the instrument, rate the extent to which each survey item represents a content area, and propose revisions if indicated).
6. Recruit participants (conduct pilot test, then the main study of instrument; obtain institutional review board approval, if indicated).
7. Evaluate validity (scale is measuring what it is intended to measure) and reliability (consistency of scores).

Source: Kalkbrenner, M. (2021). A practical guide to instrument development and score validation in social sciences research: The MEASURE Approach. *Practical Assessment, Research & Evaluation, 26*(1). https://scholarworks.umass.edu/pare/vol26/iss1/1/

Open-Ended Questions

Self-reporting, through interviews, focus groups, and free-response items on questionnaires, is often used for collecting program evaluation data. These self-reported measures are valuable to assess opinions, attitudes, beliefs, and perspectives. When designing self-reported measures, faculty should consider the use of either open- or closed-ended questions.

One type of self-report involves open-ended questions. These free-response questions do not give respondents answers to choose, but rather are phrased for respondents to explain their answers and reactions in their own words. Typically, open-ended questions begin with words such as "why" and "how" or phrases such as "tell me about...." Often they are not technically a question but a statement that asks for a response. Open-ended questions are used frequently when data cannot be placed easily into categories. For example, free-response questions may be used to assess complex and unclear issues or when answers cannot be anticipated. Although open-ended questions provide rich descriptive data, it is challenging and time-consuming for faculty to analyze and interpret responses. These were discussed in more detail in Chapter 3.

Closed-Ended Questions

Another type of self-reported measure uses a closed-ended question. Due to their structured nature, closed-ended questions limit answers as respondents are forced to choose from a set of dichotomous answers such as yes/no or true/false or from multiple

---

BOX 4.4

Examples of Program Evaluation Questions

Open-ended:
    Tell me about _____.
    How did you _____?
    How does _____ affect _____?
Closed-ended:
    How often have you _____?
    Rank the most frequently used _____.
    How many hours of _____ have you completed?
    Are you satisfied with _____?

---

responses, such as with multiple-choice questions and Likert scales. As discussed in Chapter 3, closed-ended questions may be broadly categorized as multiple-choice or ranking. Types of multiple-choice questions include nominal response, ordinal response, numeric rating, and Likert questions, and may be presented in a matrix.

Closed-ended questions might be used in program evaluation when possible answers are known, when information can be quantified, or because of their efficient method of data collection and analysis. They are usually easier to analyze, maybe more specific, and take less time for users to complete than open-ended questions. However, closed-ended questions may be more difficult to construct because the developer needs to know all the possible answers or response choices. Additionally, some critics have argued that using closed-ended questions may not represent the true feeling of respondents and may omit possible response categories. Box 4.4 offers some examples of open- and close-ended question stems for developing questions for program evaluation.

DATA COLLECTION METHODS

Regardless of the type of question, data can be obtained in a variety of formats. Some commonly used methods include surveys (completed in-person, mailed via postal mail, emailed, web-based, or completed using a mobile device); telephone surveys; face-to-face interviews; and focus groups. Each method brings unique advantages and disadvantages. Table 4.1 provides an overview of each of these methods of data collection and special considerations when using them.

Quantitative Data Collection Approaches

Faculty need to make decisions about the type of data collection method they will use for evaluation. They should consider the format that will provide the most useful data and will gather data from a sufficient number of stakeholders. Given the advantages of closed-ended questions, surveys are used frequently for collecting program evaluation data. If there are no adequate existing surveys, or if they do not meet program needs,

TABLE 4.1

Comparison of Data Collection Methods

Method	Advantages	Disadvantages	Considerations
In-person survey	Can distribute to and collect quickly and efficiently from groups. Evaluator is available to answer questions. Personal contact can positively influence response rate.	Gaining access to groups can be challenging.	Implement strategies to minimize data collector influence on responses.
Mail surveys (postal mail)	Can reach a large audience and geographic dispersion. Respondents can answer when convenient. Single evaluator can do.	Responses may be biased due to self-selection of completion. No one available to explain or answer questions. Low response rates especially if no incentives or methods to promote participation; use of advance letter/email, follow-up contacts, incentives, and variety of other procedures can increase response rates. Need to wait for responses to be returned. No control over environment when completing. Costs for duplication and mailing.	Better to use for respondents with interest in the subject. Use techniques that enhance physical appearance of survey and promote responses (e.g., prestamped return envelope). Use follow-up reminders to enhance response rates (no more than three).
Online/web-based/mobile surveys	Rapid return of responses. Real time access. Can reach large number of people. Can easily track results and respondents. Economical. Convenient for users.	Only reaches users with access to technology. May have low response rates.	Survey should be viewable from all electronic devices (mobile phones, iPad, laptops, etc.).

TABLE 4.1

Comparison of Data Collection Methods *(Continued)*

Method	Advantages	Disadvantages	Considerations
Telephone surveys	Easy to adapt to needs of respondents. Can explain questions if needed. Interviewer can probe for additional information and explanations.	Cost (human resources needed to conduct telephone survey). May have difficulty reaching participants due to call screening. People have limited time. May not have updated phone contact.	Need current phone numbers, which may not always be accessible.
Face-to-face interview	Can establish rapport with respondent. Explore topics more fully with probing and questioning techniques. Allows for use of own words and not predetermined categories. High response rates.	Time to arrange and complete interview. Interviewer can impact responses. Transcription of audio files and data analysis can be time-consuming.	Need interview guide and interviewer training.
Focus groups	Obtain opinions and viewpoints from multiple people at the same time. Allow for interaction and conversation among participants. Can explore and clarify participant responses.	Participants may be uncomfortable expressing views in group. Group members may be influenced by others in the group and strive to conform.	Consider selection of homogeneous groups. Carefully select moderator and data collection method to ensure neutrality (in person, via videoconference). Use discussion strategies to ensure participation of all members.

faculty may need to create a new survey. A few recommendations for developing a survey are found in Box 4.5.

A consideration when using a survey is the method of administration. In-person distribution of surveys often works best for students, and typically this approach improves response rates. However, surveys completed in person require a designated time for completion and may have other logistical considerations. Surveying individuals away from the nursing program's physical location may be best achieved by mail, online, or phone survey methods. Mailing surveys (via postal mail), however, is costly and relies on accurate mailing addresses. Simple steps such as a pre-letter informing participants

---

BOX 4.5

Considerations for Developing a Survey for Program Evaluation

Focus on a single item
Do not ask questions that contain multiple components
Include appropriate details
Assess relevant time period for accurate recall
Ensure statements are inclusive and without bias
Avoid negatively worded statements
Use simple clear language and familiar words understood by respondents
Spell out acronyms
Avoid jargon
Ensure that content, grammar, spelling, and punctuation are accurate
Use selective combinations of boldface type, underlining, and capitals for emphasis
Phrase in nonthreatening, straightforward, and direct manner
Ensure the content and questions apply to respondents (they have relevant experience to answer)
Make choices mutually exclusive and not overlapping
Have items reviewed by others prior to use
Pretest and pilot test newly developed items

---

about an upcoming survey and its importance and including a self-addressed pre-stamped envelope can improve response rates for mailed surveys (Dillman, Smythe, & Christian, 2014). Online surveys (with a link sent electronically, on a web page, or a mobile device) have become the predominant method of administration for surveys because of their ease, opportunity for a quick response, and low cost (Saleh & Bista, 2017). Online surveys, however, have a lower response rate than in-person administration and when mailed. Short and concise surveys with a limited number, if any, of open-ended items increase response rates for online surveys (Saleh & Bista, 2017). Other strategies to encourage responses to an online survey are provided in Box 4.6. Potential respondents can

---

BOX 4.6

Strategies to Improve Response Rates with Online Surveys

1. Have a person well known to the participants distribute the survey or include a request from them to complete it.
2. In the invitation with the survey, explain the importance of the survey, include the approximate time it will take for completion, and ensure anonymity for respondents (do not request information that could identify respondents) and confidentiality of responses.
3. Keep the survey short and concise with no or limited open-ended items.
4. Consider including an incentive for survey completion.
5. Send at least one, but not more than three, reminders to complete the survey.
6. Consider timing for distribution of the survey.

Adapted from Saleh, A., & Bista, K. (2017). Examining factors impacting online survey response rates in educational research: Perceptions of graduate students. *Journal of MultiDisciplinary Evaluation, 13*(29), 63–74. https://journals.sfu.ca/jmde/index.php/jmde_1/article/view/487

be alerted to an upcoming survey and delivery method by email or using Facebook or another social media platform.

Sampling and sample size are other considerations when using survey methods. Will convenience or probability sampling methods be used? Should all students, graduates, or other individuals or groups be invited to participate? Regardless of the survey method, faculty should consider varied alternatives and have a rationale for the choices made.

Qualitative Data Collection Approaches

There are a variety of data collection methods that use open-ended questions and employ traditional qualitative research methods. Three commonly used qualitative methods for program evaluation are interviews, focus groups, and ePortfolios.

Interviews

Individual interviews allow nurse educators to elicit rich descriptions about the school, nursing program, student and faculty perceptions, and other areas to answer the evaluation questions and provide data about the program. With an interview, the evaluator also can engage in an in-depth conversation about issues or problems. The interview should be guided by carefully constructed questions and conducted in a mutually convenient private location. With the availability of technology, such as videoconferencing, interviews can now be easily conducted from a remote location. Many interviewers use a semi-structured interview guide to direct key elements of the conversation, with prompts to probe for additional information. Interviewers can take notes during or after the session to aid the recall of key aspects of the interview. Interviews can be audio recorded followed by line-by-line transcription to provide a verbatim record for data analysis. Data analysis should yield common or reoccurring findings.

Focus Groups

Focus groups, another form of qualitative data collection, consist of a guided conversation by a trained facilitator with a group of participants. Using a carefully constructed interview guide and encouraging interaction, the facilitator elicits the sharing of views, feelings, attitudes, and experiences that leads to a collective understanding of a topic and can be used to identify important themes (Krueger & Casey, 2015; Rossi, Lipsey, & Henry, 2019; Tritter & Landstad, 2020). Box 4.7 provides some general guidelines for use of focus groups and some sample questions. The purpose of the focus group is not to reach consensus among the participants but to seek opinions and viewpoints. The facilitator creates an atmosphere that encourages interaction and dynamic exchange among participants. Depending on the targeted group and topic, the exact size of the focus group can vary, but in general, small groups of participants, usually five to eight, are recommended.

Faculty planning focus groups need to make a number of decisions about the data collection approach. They should carefully create open-ended questions that lead to conversational discussions about the topic. Those participating in a focus group need to have experience or familiarity with the topic. For example, selecting first-semester students to engage in a focus group about their clinical experiences, when they have

---

BOX 4.7

Focus Group Guide and Sample Questions

Welcome participants

Explain purpose and structure of focus group

Ensure privacy and confidentiality

Begin with opening question or statement that can be answered by all and engages all participants
   (e.g., tell us what program you are enrolled in)

Ask key questions, for example:
   What do you think of ...?
   What do you like best about ...?
   What do you like least about ...?
   How has the program helped you to develop ...? In what ways?
   How could the program be improved?
   Think back to ... experience. What was that experience like for you?

Allow participants to offer differing points of view or confirm what has already been said

Use pauses to allow participation

Probe for additional information by using statements such as:
   Can you give an example?
   Would you explain what you mean by ...?

Conclude the group by asking about any missing information and thank participants

---

only participated in a few days of clinical learning, would not provide quality data. Conversely, inviting senior students who have participated in numerous clinical learning opportunities to participate in a focus group to discuss their clinical learning and sites would lead to a much richer and more descriptive conversation.

The identification and selection of participants is another important issue that can impact data collection and quality. A challenge that many focus group planners encounter involves scheduling when the focus group will meet. Faculty should consider the pool of participants and their schedule demands and plan for focus groups that are conveniently scheduled, such as close to students' class time. Or, if planning a focus group for alumni, faculty might consider when potential participants would be available, such as during a time when alumni return to the school of nursing. Instead of groups meeting in person, online focus groups are being used increasingly (Lobe & Morgan, 2021). Morrison et al. (2020) described using web conference technology for data collection with focus groups across Canada.

Unlike questionnaires that can be completed quickly, focus groups require more time for participation, and faculty might consider offering incentives to encourage participation. Depending on the budget and purchasing restrictions, small tokens of appreciation can be provided. When carefully planned and executed, focus groups can provide valuable data for program evaluation.

ePortfolios

Many nursing programs use electronic portfolios or ePortfolios to document students' achievement of competencies and program outcomes (Willmarth-Stec & Beery, 2015).

Traditionally, educational portfolios were a collection of paper-based student arti-facts (documents) such as papers, concept maps, journals, and evaluation materials. The materials were assembled to document growth or to provide a collection of best works as evidence for evaluation in a course or program (Oermann & Gaberson, 2021). With changes in student demographics, advances in technology, and the need for port-folio portability and accessibility of portfolio materials, many nursing programs have shifted to ePortfolios (Oermann & Gaberson, 2021; Sabio et al., 2020; Willmarth-Stec & Beery, 2015). The purpose of the ePortfolio is the same as the traditional, hard copy portfolio; how-ever, diverse multimedia materials such as video, audio, and other digital artifacts can be included.

Faculty face a number of challenges when using ePortfolios for nursing program evaluation. One challenge is the time needed for creation, orientation, and evaluation of portfolio materials. Students need orientation to the ePortfolio requirements, clear directions about the purpose, and guidelines for developing it. Additionally, decisions are needed as to the evaluation of the ePortfolio and careful construction of scoring rubrics, if used for the evaluation.

Existing Assessment Tools

Assessments made at the end of a program of study, sometimes referred to as exit examinations or exit evaluations, provide valuable information that can guide program decisions. Faculty may feel overwhelmed in creating a survey that gathers comprehen-sive end-of-program information and yields meaningful data and may decide to use existing data collection tools rather than creating their own.

There are a number of existing assessment tools that are available for this purpose. For example, Skyfactor Benchworks (2021) offers graduating student, alumni, and employer surveys for an associate degree in nursing, bachelor of science in nursing, master of science in nursing, and DNP programs. Surveys are mapped to the standards of each of the accrediting organizations in nursing. Nationally or commercially devel-oped tools have a number of advantages. They are designed by experts in test con-struction who have access to significant resources, are tested with a broad sample of participants in diverse settings, and provide benchmarking data for schools. Faculty should carefully review existing tools, determine their alignment with the program out-comes, and evaluate if the tools will meet their data collection and program evalua-tion needs. Faculty also should consider student demographics, costs, availability, and delivery of products when making a decision to use existing tools.

CAPTURING DATA FROM KEY STAKEHOLDERS

Program evaluation plans typically include data collection from a variety of key stake-holders. Obviously, a major stakeholder is the nursing student. Many data collection strategies will involve soliciting student input and feedback throughout the program. Accessing and gathering data from students is not usually difficult as they are easily accessible and frequently willing to provide the needed information. It also is impor-tant that data come from other key stakeholders including graduates, preceptors, and employers; however, gathering data from these groups can be challenging. Some schools of nursing use advisory groups to provide input about the program and assist with strategic visioning and planning. If the school has academic partnerships, these relationships can be used as a source of program evaluation data.

Technology Use

Technology such as Facebook, Twitter, and other social media platforms provides creative data collection opportunities. Virtual digital platforms can be used to alert students, alumni, and community stakeholders about a survey from the school of nursing to recruit participants and engage in conversations about health and research topics (Forgasz et al., 2018; Patten et al., 2021). Professional networking sites, such as LinkedIn, also have potential for recruiting participants for surveys and eliciting feedback about the nursing program.

Faculty considering using these approaches for recruitment and data collection should realize the limitations of the technology for program evaluation. Only those with access to the social media site can be reached; it is reasonable to assume that not all alumni and other stakeholders are represented on social media. Additionally, faculty need the technical expertise to set up profiles and groups and post messages using these networking websites.

Technology, such as videoconferencing, can be used to interact with alumni, clinical partners, and community stakeholders to provide input for nursing program evaluation. Since faculty may have difficulty gathering data from these groups due to time demands, scheduling constraints, distance, and costs, alternative methods using technology are valuable. A variety of videoconferencing options such as Zoom (https://zoom.us/) or Microsoft® Teams (https://www.microsoft.com/en-us/microsoft-teams/group-chat-software) may assist in connecting with key program stakeholders and others. Some of these communication platforms offer recording options to document a record of the videoconference session. Before implementing this approach for data collection, though, it is important to carefully select the platform that will be most effective for meeting program and participant needs. Faculty should practice with the equipment and become familiar with it before using it for formal data collection. Costs also need to be considered. Some videoconferencing programs are free while others that offer deluxe options or special features have a cost. Ease of use, quality of audio and video, and the need for special equipment such as a webcam are other factors to consider.

ENSURING STANDARDS IN PROGRAM EVALUATION

Regardless of the methods used for data collection, faculty need to follow professional and ethical practices to ensure quality data and to protect participants. The Joint Committee on Standards for Educational Evaluation (2021) provides educators with standards on utility (the extent to which stakeholders find the evaluation processes and products valuable in meeting their needs); feasibility (effectiveness of the evaluation); propriety (proper, fair, legal, right, and just evaluations); accuracy (dependability and truthfulness of evaluation findings and judgments); and accountability (evaluation focused on program improvement and accountability).

One important aspect of collecting program evaluation data that administrators, faculty, and others involved in the evaluation should consider is confidentiality of information. Sensitive information should be stored in secure locations. If electronic data are collected, it should require a password to access, and firewalls should be established to prevent unauthorized access. Since interviewers and facilitators of focus groups will know the identity of participants, care should be taken to ensure confidentiality of data and protection of participant identity. Using pseudonyms or code numbers rather than names is one strategy that can be used to de-identify participants and enhance protection. Faculty reviewing and reporting data need to take measures to aggregate information and report group data.

The nursing program should establish guidelines or procedures for the use and access of all evaluation data. Collected data and participant information should be kept in secure electronic files. Faculty must adhere to all applicable privacy laws such as the Family Educational Rights and Privacy Act (U. S. Department of Education, 2021). Programs also should discuss how long they will retain evaluation data. Another consideration presented in national testing standards involves test security and protection of test copyrights. If using existing data collection tools, faculty should obtain copyright permission and comply with administration guidelines for use of these items, ensuring security of materials (American Educational Research Association, American Psychological Association, and National Council on Measurement in Education, 2014).

Faculty involved in collecting program evaluation data from students, faculty, and others should submit for review and approval by the Institutional Review Board (IRB) before beginning data collection if they intend on sharing the data for scholarly purposes, such as in professional presentations, publications, and reports (Oermann et al., 2021). The IRB will likely indicate the study is exempt because there is minimal risk and may be part of normal educational practices. Since guidelines and standards for reviews can vary and change over time, it is always advisable to consult institutional policies and local IRBs to ensure guidelines are followed. Regardless, if a formal IRB proposal is required, faculty should adhere to the same ethical principles of beneficence, respect, and justice when collecting data for program evaluation purposes as for research. Participation should be voluntary and not onerous, the benefits of participation should outweigh the risks, participants' identities should remain confidential, and data should be protected.

When conducting program evaluation activities, it is important to prevent bias and ensure uniform assessment approaches are used. Faculty should take steps to promote nondiscriminatory inclusive sampling and objective reporting. Data collection steps and analysis of the results should be transparent and clear for reviewers.

Summary

Program evaluation is a complex process involving many decisions. Faculty should consider data sources, psychometric issues, the type of data needed, and the best tools and methods for obtaining this information. Determining how to capture data from key stakeholders while ensuring adherence to appropriate standards is also part of the choices that faculty make as part of the evaluation of nursing programs. Making good choices about the data collection process can lead to quality evaluation data that serve as the basis for well-informed evidence-based decisions for nursing programs.

References

American Educational Research Association, American Psychological Association, and National Council on Measurement in Education. (2014). *Standards for educational and psychological testing*. https://www.testing-standards.net/uploads/7/6/6/4/76643089/standards_2014edition.pdf.

Brookhart, S. M., & Nitko, A. J. (2019). *Educational assessment of students* (9th ed.). Pearson Education.

Dillman, D. A., Smythe, J. D., & Christian, L. M. (2014). *Internet, mail, and mixed-mode surveys: The tailored design method* (4th ed.). John Wiley & Sons.

Forgasz, H., Tan, H., Leder, G., & McLeod, A. (2018). Enhancing survey participation: Facebook advertisements for recruitment in educational research. *International Journal of Research & Method in Education, 41*(3), 257–270. https://doi.org/10.1080/1743727X.2017.1295939

Joint Committee on Standards for Educational Evaluation. (2021). *Program evaluation standards*. https://evaluationstandards.org/program/

Kalkbrenner, M. (2021). A practical guide to instrument development and score validation in social sciences research: The MEASURE approach. *Practical Assessment, Research & Evaluation, 26*(1). https://scholarworks.umass.edu/pare/vol26/iss1/1/

Krueger, R. A., & Casey, M. A. (2015). *Focus groups: A practical guide for applied research*. SAGE Publications Inc.

Le, A., Han, B. H., & Palamar, J. J. (2021). When national drug surveys "take too long": An examination of who is at risk for survey fatigue. *Drug and Alcohol Dependence, 225*, 108769. https://doi.org/10.1016/j.drugalcdep.2021.108769

Lewallen, L. P. (2015). Practical strategies for nursing education program evaluation. *Journal of Professional Nursing, 31*(2), 133–140. doi: 10.1016/j.profnurs.2014.09.002

Lobe, B., & Morgan, D. L. (2021). Assessing the effectiveness of video-based interviewing: A systematic comparison of video-conferencing based dyadic interviews and focus groups. *International Journal of Social Research Methodology, 24*(3), 301–312. https://doi.org/10.1080/13645579.2020.1785763

McNeish, D. (2018). Thanks coefficient alpha, we'll take it from here. *Psychological Methods, 23*(3), 412–433. https://doi.org/10.1037/met0000144

Morrison, D., Lichtenwald, K., & Tang, R. (2020). Extending the online focus group method using web-based conferencing to explore older adults online learning. *International Journal of Research & Method in Education, 43*(1), 78–92. https://doi.org/10.1080/1743727X.2019.1594183

Oermann, M. H., Barton, A., Yoder-Wise, P. S., & Morton, P. G. (2021). Research in nursing education and the institutional review board/ethics committee. *Journal of Professional Nursing, 37*(2), 342–347. https://doi.org/10.1016/j.profnurs.2021.01.003

Oermann, M. H., & Gaberson, K. B. (2021). *Evaluation and testing in nursing education* (6th ed.). Springer.

Patten, C. A., Balls-Berry, J. J. E., Cohen, E. L., Brockman, T. A., Valdez Soto, M., West, I. W., Cha, J., Zavala Rocha, M. G., & Eder, M. M. (2021). Feasibility of a virtual Facebook community platform for engagement on health research. *Journal of Clinical and Translational Science, 5*(1), e85–e85. https://doi.org/10.1017/cts.2021.12

Rossi, P. H., Lipsey, M. W., & Henry, G. T. (2019). *Evaluation: A systematic approach* (8th ed.). SAGE Publications Inc.

Sabio, C., Chen, J., Moxley, E. A., Taylor, L., Kuchinski, A. M., & Peters, B. T. (2020). Improving portfolio assessment: Addressing challenges in transition to eportfolio. *Journal of Nursing Education, 59*(12), 705708. https://doi.org/10.3928/01484834-20201118-09

Saleh, A., & Bista, K. (2017). Examining factors impacting online survey response rates in educational research: Perceptions of graduate students. *Journal of MultiDisciplinary Evaluation, 13*(29), 63–74. https://journals.sfu.ca/jmde/index.php/jmde_1/article/view/487

Skyfactor Benchworks™. (2021). Nursing education. Accessed January 2, 2022. https://www.skyfactor.com/academics/nursing-education/

Stewart, J., Joyce, J., Haines, M., Yanoski, D., Gagnon, D., Luke, K., Rhoads, C., & Germeroth, C. (2021) *Program Evaluation Toolkit: Quick Start Guide* (REL 2022–112) U. S. Department of Education, Institute of Education Sciences, National Center for Education Evaluation and Regional Assistance, Regional Educational Laboratory Central. http://ies ed gov/ncee/edlabs

Taber, K. S. (2018). The use of Cronbach's alpha when developing and reporting research instruments in science education. *Research in Science Education, 48*(6), 1273–1296. https://doi.org/10.1007/s11165-016-9602-2

Tritter, J. Q., & Landstad, B. J. (2020). Focus groups. In C. Pope & N. Mays (Eds.), *Qualitative research in health care* (4th ed., pp. 57–66). Wiley. https://doi.org/10.1002/9781119410867.ch5

U.S. Department of Education. Protecting student privacy. Accessed December 28, 2021. https://studentprivacy.ed.gov/Apps

Willmarth-Stec, M., & Beery, T. (2015). Operationalizing the student electronic portfolio for doctoral nursing education. *Nurse Educator, 40*(5), 263–265. https://doi.org/10.1097/nne.0000000000000161

5

The Accreditation Process in Nursing Education

Teresa Shellenbarger, PhD, RN, CNE, CNEcl, ANEF

The nursing workforce in the United States (US) depends on nursing education programs to produce an adequate pool of competent nursing graduates who are prepared to meet health care demands. Since no single authority exercises control over post-secondary education in the US, accreditation serves as the primary means of communicating educational quality. This chapter describes the purpose of higher education (post-secondary) accreditation in the US, types of accreditation, and typical program elements represented in accreditation standards for nursing education. An overview of the accreditation process is also provided. The relationship among program evaluation, continuous quality improvement, and the accreditation process is emphasized throughout the chapter.

PURPOSE OF ACCREDITATION

Accreditation of US higher education institutions and programs offers a form of educational quality assurance. The external review process associated with accreditation helps protect the public while indicating that a program or school meets a minimum level of acceptable quality. In the US, the first voluntary association that offered peer review of programs occurred in the late 19th century (Hegji, 2020). Nursing began educational accreditation activities in 1938 when the National League for Nursing Education (NLNE), later known as the National League for Nursing, initiated accreditation for nursing education (National League for Nursing, 2021). Since then, nursing programs have continued to engage in accreditation activities to ensure nursing program quality.

Accreditation is a voluntary process that nursing programs frequently pursue. Achieving nursing program accreditation ensures accountability to stakeholders and assists in the protection of the public. Attaining accreditation offers a distinction of program effectiveness and quality while also offering additional benefits for students, alumni, and other stakeholders. Box 5.1 provides some of the benefits associated with accreditation. Many nursing education programs seek accreditation for participation in federal programs and for gaining access to federal and state funding. Some nursing

---

BOX 5.1

Benefits of Accreditation

Serves as evidence of quality assurance to stakeholders such as students and the public
Grants institutions eligibility to access federal and state funding
Offers evidence of quality to community members such as employers or donors
Facilitates students' academic credit transfer between institutions

---

Source: Council for Higher Education Accreditation. (n.d.). *About accreditation.* https://www.chea.org/about-accreditation

programs require graduate program applicants to have completed prior education from an accredited program. For example, graduate nursing programs may not admit students unless they have graduated from an accredited prelicensure program. Employers may also decline to hire nurses who have not graduated from accredited nursing programs, and some health care agencies will only provide clinical learning experiences for students enrolled in accredited programs. Institutions and programs participate in the accreditation process for a variety of reasons, but ultimately they participate to demonstrate program quality to the community, such as employers or donors, and students enrolled in their program.

It is important to understand the distinctions between accreditation and regulatory authority, as they are different and independent processes (Kremer & Horton, 2020). For example, state boards of nursing are regulatory bodies that hold the authority to regulate both nursing practice and nursing education. Nursing programs cannot operate without state authorization granted to them by the appropriate state board of nursing. Some state boards of nursing term this authorization *approval,* while other state boards of nursing use the term *accreditation*. Regardless of whether the term is approval or accreditation, the regulatory authorization granted by state boards of nursing is different from that of the accreditation status granted by national nursing accrediting agencies. Boards of nursing grant authorization for nursing programs to operate because they hold state regulatory responsibility for protecting the public's welfare, health, and safety (National Council of State Boards of Nursing [NCSBN], 2021b). Nursing programs must comply with the regulations set forth by the state board of the state (or states) within which they operate, or the board of nursing has the authority to suspend or close the program's operation (NCSBN, 2020). In contrast, accreditation by a national nursing accrediting agency is a voluntary, nongovernmental process, which nursing programs opt to pursue as a public mark of quality assurance. While accrediting agencies can deny or revoke the program's accreditation if the program does not meet the accreditation standards, they do not have the authority to suspend program operations or close the program.

More than 20 state nursing regulatory bodies require national nursing accreditation for prelicensure nursing programs (NCSBN, 2021a). Thus, while the accreditation process is described as voluntary, it is increasingly important that institutions and programs participate in the process. Participating in the accreditation process requires the institution or program to formally engage in a systematic evaluation process, identify strengths and areas for improvement, and contribute to ongoing quality improvement efforts.

ACCREDITATION AND ROLE OF THE US DEPARTMENT OF EDUCATION

The US Department of Education (USDE) is not directly involved in the accreditation of post-secondary institutions or programs. The USDE recognizes accrediting agencies that are considered reliable authorities for setting standards and evaluating the quality of the institutions and programs they accredit. Federal law requires the USDE to maintain a published national listing of all institutional and programmatic accrediting agencies recognized by the USDE (USDE, 2021).

The USDE plays an essential role in recognizing accrediting agencies. Seeking recognition from the USDE is a voluntary activity for accrediting agencies. The USDE will only recognize those agencies that apply and meet criteria found in a published set of standards (USDE, 2020). The USDE specifies that accrediting agencies must complete various actions that demonstrate they consistently apply and enforce accreditation standards. They must use those standards to assess student achievement, and, as applicable, include assessment of course completion, the passing of licensure examinations, and job placement rates. The accrediting agency must evaluate curriculum, faculty, facilities, and fiscal and administrative capacity. Lastly, agencies must meet operational procedures and follow due process procedures (Hegji, 2020).

Title IV and Accreditation

The USDE specifically recognizes some accrediting agencies as "gatekeepers" of Title IV funds. Title IV of the Higher Education Act of 1965, as amended, addresses the federal student financial assistance programs administered by the USDE. To be considered eligible for Title IV funding, institutions need to meet three criteria, known as the *program integrity triad:* (1) state authorization, (2) accreditation by a USDE recognized accrediting agency, and (3) verification by the USDE of the institution's eligibility to manage federal financial aid programs (Hegji, 2020).

Therefore, any post-secondary institution or program wanting to administer federally-funded financial assistance to its students must be accredited by an agency that the USDE recognizes for Title IV gatekeeping purposes. For most post-secondary institutions and the associated academic programs, this requirement is met through accreditation by a regional or national institutional accreditor. However, in some cases, the nursing program may be administratively housed in institutions that are not eligible for regional or national institutional accreditation. In nursing education, this most commonly happens in practical/vocational and diploma nursing programs if they are located within technical institutions or hospitals. Such programs must then seek accreditation from a programmatic accreditor recognized by the USDE for Title IV purposes. The only programmatic accreditor holding this recognition in nursing is the Accreditation Commission for Education in Nursing (ACEN).

TYPES OF ACCREDITATION

There are two types of accreditation in higher education: institutional and programmatic accreditation (Hegji, 2020). Institutional accreditation is awarded to all aspects of the entire college or university and includes all programs. Programmatic accreditation,

---

BOX 5.2

US Regional Accrediting Agencies

Accrediting Commission for Community and Junior Colleges (ACCJC), Western Association of Schools and Colleges
Middle States Commission on Higher Education (MSCHE)
New England Commission of Higher Education (NECHE)
The Higher Learning Commission (HLC)
Northwest Commission on Colleges and Universities (NWCCU)
Southern Association of Colleges and Schools, Commission on Colleges (SACSCOC)
Western Association of Schools and Colleges (WASC), Senior Colleges, and University Commission Colleges

---

Source: Council for Higher Education Accreditation. (2021). *Directory of CHEA-recognized organizations.* https://www.chea.org/sites/default/files/other-content/directory-CHEA-recognized-orgs_105.pdf

also known as specialized accreditation, is granted to schools, programs, or departments, and is usually focused on a single discipline.

Institutional Accrediting Agencies

Institutional accrediting agencies grant accreditation to colleges and universities. There are two primary categories of institutional accreditors: regional and national. Seven regional accrediting agencies that are Title IV gatekeepers of federal funds operate throughout the US. Box 5.2 provides a list of regional accreditors in the US. Regional accrediting agencies accredit private and public, 2- and 4-year degree-granting colleges and universities that are primarily nonprofit. As of February 2017, these regional accreditors accredited 3524 institutions (Hegji, 2020).

The second category of institutional accrediting agencies is primarily faith-based or career-related agencies. They accredit mainly proprietary and career-based single-purpose institutions. As of February 2017, the career-related accrediting agencies accredited approximately 1787 institutions across the US (Hegji, 2020).

Achieving institutional accreditation benefits the institution's academic programs. The public mark of quality that institutional accreditation conveys is an assurance that the institution has processes in place that enable it to meet established standards, maintain fiscal stability, employ qualified faculty, offer federally funded student financial assistance, have adequate student support services, and provide quality curricula. Having such solid institutional infrastructures in place, as indicated by achieving accreditation, assists programs to leverage the resources of the institution to maintain quality and recruit students to their programs.

Programmatic Accreditation

Programmatic accrediting agencies, also known as specialized accrediting agencies, review programs rather than institutions. Academic programs such as nursing and other health professions, law, business, and engineering are examples of specific programs that are accredited by programmatic accreditors. These programs may be public or private, nonprofit, or for-profit in status.

In the nursing profession, three programmatic accrediting agencies accredit nursing programs. Historically, the National League for Nursing (NLN) was the first nursing education program accreditor in the nursing profession. The NLN's accrediting activities are currently carried out by the Commission for Nursing Education Accreditation (CNEA). Established in 2013 as an autonomous accreditation division of the NLN, CNEA accredits all types of nursing programs, including practical/vocational, diploma, associate, bachelor, master's, and clinical doctorate programs. The CNEA received recognition as a programmatic accreditor by the USDE in 2021.

A second USDE-recognized programmatic accreditor in nursing is the Commission on Collegiate Nursing Education (CCNE). The CCNE is the autonomous accreditation arm of the American Association of Colleges of Nursing. The CCNE accredits baccalaureate and higher degree nursing programs and has conducted accreditation activities since 1998 (CCNE, 2018a).

The third programmatic accreditor in nursing education is the Accreditation Commission for Education in Nursing (ACEN), formerly known as the NLNAC. The ACEN accredits all types of nursing programs and is the only nursing program accreditor recognized by the USDE as a Title IV gatekeeper for nursing programs requiring this function.

There are also specialty accreditors in nursing education. The Council on Accreditation (COA) of Nurse Anesthesia is the accrediting agency for nursing programs that prepare nurse anesthetists. The Accreditation Commission for Midwifery Education (ACME) accredits nursing programs that educate nurse-midwives. The USDE recognizes both agencies.

Nursing programs can select the nursing accrediting agency for their accreditation needs. Some programs opt to be accredited by more than one agency. The program's administrators and faculty need to carefully consider which accreditation agency best aligns with its mission and goals before determining the agency that is the best fit for the program. While accreditation standards and policies can be similar, the values and philosophical approach to the accreditation process may vary among agencies.

ACCREDITATION STANDARDS

The agency accreditation standards provide direction for the accreditation process. Accreditation standards are applied at the institutional and program levels. At the program level, accreditation standards reflect the professional standards, values, curricular concepts, and educational outcomes espoused by the profession. As such, accreditation standards are set by the profession and include input from various stakeholders, such as educators, practice partners, and the public.

In addition to any accreditation elements that the profession identifies as essential to ensuring quality, the USDE has identified some common elements that USDE-recognized accrediting agencies are expected to include in their accreditation standards for institutions and programs. Box 5.3 provides a list of these expected standards of elements. Because of these USDE expectations, the accreditation standards of many accrediting agencies include a common set of standards and criteria, which are similar

---

BOX 5.3

Elements of Accreditation Standards Required by the US Department of Education

Successful student achievement as related to institution/program mission, including course completion rates, licensure/certification rates, job placement rates
Curricula
Faculty
Facilities, equipment, and supplies
Fiscal/administrative capacity
Student support services
Policies regarding advertising and publications (recruiting, admissions, grading, etc.)
Description of program length and objectives of the degree credentials offered[a]
Record of complaints received from students
Evidence of compliance with Title IV of the Higher Education Act[a]

---

[a]Expected of accrediting agencies recognized by the USDE for Title IV gatekeeping purposes.

Source: *Accreditation and preaccreditation standards, 34 C.F.R. § 602.16* (November 1, 2019). U.S. Government Publishing Office. https://www.ecfr.gov/current/title-34/subtitle-B/chapter-VI/part-602/subpart-B

in nature and foci. The specific evidence and indicators of quality for each standard can vary, as well as the labeling of the standards; however, all USDE-recognized agencies must include these core elements. Table 5.1 lists the accreditation standards for ACEN, CCNE, and CNEA and the specific standards that align with the USDE guidelines. The USDE expectations for accreditation standards are described further in the following paragraphs.

Successful Student Achievement

Accreditation standards are expected to address student achievement of program outcomes that align with the institution's mission. Specific areas that need to be addressed include student success on licensure and certification examinations, program completion rates, and employment rates. Programs are also expected to have an assessment and evaluation plan that fosters the collection and analysis of data designed to measure student achievement of expected outcomes. Programs will use the feedback from data analysis for program improvement purposes (USDE, 2020).

There are differences among the nursing accreditation agencies in how these outcomes are gathered and reported by programs, as well as the specificity of expected performance outcomes. For example, the CCNE (2018b) prescribes that employment rates, collected at any time within 12 months of program completion, be 70% or higher. Conversely, the ACEN (2020a) does not set a performance benchmark but allows faculty to determine the expected level of achievement for job placement. They expect programs to provide data from at least the three most recent reporting years. The CNEA (2021) also allows programs to set their own performance benchmarks but specifies that data should be collected within six to 12 months of graduation, and programs must

TABLE 5.1

Accreditation Standards for ACEN, CCNE, and CNEA Aligned with USDE Required Educational Standards

USDE Required Educational Standards	ACEN	CCNE	CNEA
Student Achievement	Standard 6 Outcomes	Standard IV Program Effectiveness: Assessment and Achievement of Program Outcomes	Standard I: Culture of Excellence–Program Outcomes
Curricula	Standard 4 Curriculum	Standard III Program Quality: Curriculum and Teaching/Learning Practices	Standard V: Culture of Learning and Diversity–Curriculum and Evaluation Processes
Faculty	Standard 1 Mission and Administrative Capacity	Standard II Program Quality: Institutional Commitment and Resources	Standard III: Culture of Excellence and Caring–Faculty
	Standard 2 Faculty and Staff	Standard IV Program Effectiveness: Assessment and Achievement of Program Outcomes	
Facilities Equipment and Supplies	Standard 5 Resources	Standard II Program Quality: Institutional Commitment and Resources	Standard II: Culture of Integrity and Accountability–Mission, Governance, and Resources
Fiscal and Administrative Capacity	Standard 1 Mission and Administrative Capacity	Standard II Program Quality: Institutional Commitment and Resources	Standard II: Culture of Integrity and Accountability–Mission, Governance, and Resources
	Standard 5 Resources		
Student Support Services	Standard 3 Students	Standard II Program Quality: Institutional Commitment and Resources	Standard IV: Culture of Excellence and Caring–Students
Policies About Advertising and Publications	Standard 3 Students	Standard II Program Quality: Institutional Commitment and Resources	Standard IV: Culture of Excellence and Caring–Students
		Standard I Program Quality: Mission and Governance	
Records of Student Complaints	Standard 3 Students	Standard I Program Quality: Mission and Governance	Standard IV: Culture of Excellence and Caring–Students

Note: ACEN, Accreditation Commission for Education in Nursing; CCNE, Commission on Collegiate Nursing Education; CNEA, Commission for Nursing Education Accreditation; USDE, US Department of Education.

Source: ACEN. (2020a). *Accreditation manual: Section III: Standards and criteria.* https://www.acenursing.org/Resources-for-Nursing-Programs/sc2017-B.pdf; CCNE. (2018b). *Standards for accreditation of baccalaureate and graduate nursing programs.* https://www.aacnnursing.org/Portals/42/CCNE/PDF/Standards-Final-2018.pdf; CNEA. (2021). *Accreditation standards for nursing education programs.* https://cnea.nln.org/standards-of-accreditation

provide trended data from three academic years. Even though all accrediting agencies require reporting about these program outcomes, faculty are encouraged to become familiar with the specific reporting requirements for the selected accrediting agency as they do vary among the nursing accrediting agencies.

Curriculum

Standards related to the program curricula are expected to address the specific degree level of the program and be correlated with the institution's mission. The curriculum of distance education programs should be similar to what is delivered on campus. In addition, standards of accreditation are expected to address appropriate sequencing of courses, incorporation of educational concepts, and relevance of courses related to the major. Course objectives are expected to be specified (USDE, 2020). Areas commonly included as part of curriculum evaluation include the inclusion of professional standards in courses and throughout the curriculum, clinical or simulation learning experiences, course sequencing, course syllabi, and content in courses that reflect current nursing knowledge and relevant professional issues.

The nursing accrediting agencies also vary in the specificity of some of the curriculum areas. Both the CNEA (2021) and ACEN (2020a) state that programs must incorporate professional standards and guidelines, but they allow the program to self-identify relevant materials. In contrast, CCNE requires specific standards and guidelines for use in the curriculum. In their accreditation standards, they indicate the documents that must be incorporated. For example, baccalaureate programs must incorporate the AACN essentials into the curriculum. Each program level has specific standards they must include (CCNE, 2018b).

Faculty

Faculty must have the requisite knowledge necessary to teach the courses they have been assigned and demonstrate the appropriate education and experience to qualify them for their teaching role. Programs may provide data such as faculty licensure, certification, educational preparation, and continuing education activities. Standards are expected to address the number of faculty required to meet the program's mission adequately. Programs may describe student-to-faculty ratios for courses. Criteria related to faculty development and evaluation are other key elements expected to be addressed in this standard (USDE, 2020). Programs may also discuss faculty expectations and provide information about teaching, advisement, scholarship, and service activities of faculty.

Facilities, Equipment, and Supplies

Demonstrating that the program has the resources necessary to achieve its mission and goals is essential for sustaining quality. The resources include a budget that is sufficient to maintain and expand, as needed, the physical facilities for classrooms and laboratories; instructional equipment and supplies; and technical infrastructure that is sufficient to provide student support services and deliver distance education (USDE, 2020). Evidence to support the achievement of standards related to this area may include budget tables, resource assessments such as inventories of laboratory equipment, or physical facilities used by the program. Related resources that support student learning, such as library or instructional resources, may comprise another critical example of support related to facilities, equipment, and supplies.

Fiscal and Administrative Capacity

Expectations for this standard are that the program can demonstrate financial and administrative stability and adequate staff to implement the program's mission. Program administrators must have clearly defined roles and responsibilities and be appropriately qualified for their position (USDE, 2020). Programs may provide evidence of capacity in this area through administrator job descriptions or budget tables.

Student Support Services

Standards related to student support services are expected to address the adequacy and effectiveness of the support services in helping students achieve academic success. Such support services may include having access to financial aid, academic advising, career guidance, health, personal counseling, and other services. Maintaining the confidentiality and security of student records is another accreditation expectation (USDE, 2020). Programs can provide information about available student support services.

Policies about Advertising and Publications

Being accurate and clear in advertising and publications when communicating with program stakeholders is an important public demonstration of program integrity. The USDE expects that accrediting agencies will have standards that address the clarity and accuracy of the program's policies and practices related to recruiting and admissions, grading policies, and the publication of catalogs, academic calendars, recruitment materials, and other program documents (USDE, 2020). Programs will be expected to show copies of written materials shared with stakeholders to allow for an analysis of this information.

Description of Program Length and Degree Credentials

Accrediting agencies that serve as Title IV gatekeepers are expected to have standards that address the usual program length and credit hours. Since these programs serve as financial aid gatekeepers for student financial aid, they need a means of assuring that students are enrolled in programs that have a curriculum and required credit hours that are congruent with program type and degree credentials. Programs not recognized for Title IV gatekeeping are not required to address this element in their standards (USDE, 2020).

Record of Complaints Received from Students

As one means of protecting student interests, it is expected that accrediting agencies will have standards that address formal student complaints and how the program manages them. It is an expectation that programs maintain records of student complaints, including documentation of how the complaints have been resolved, and provide this information as part of the program review (USDE, 2020).

Evidence of Compliance with Title IV of Higher Education Act

In keeping with their responsibilities as Title IV gatekeepers, all accrediting agencies that have been recognized as such by the USDE are expected to have standards related to the institution's or program's compliance with Title IV regulations. Areas of compliance would include compliance audits, loan default rates, and other required reports requested by the USDE (USDE, 2020).

To summarize, accreditation standards serve as the foundation for the accreditation process. Standards developed by accrediting agencies are derived from a profession's standards, values, curricular concepts, and expected educational outcomes. Additionally, the USDE has a set of expectations for all accrediting agencies recognized by the USDE. To achieve accreditation, institutions and programs must demonstrate their ability to meet the identified standards. They demonstrate their compliance by participating in the external and public peer review accreditation process. An important part of accreditation is demonstrating evidence of these specific items and the program's focus on quality improvement. The program is expected to gather data on an ongoing basis and use that information for program improvement. With input from various stakeholders such as students, faculty, alumni, practice partners, and the community, the program can decide what is working and what areas need to be changed. This continuous quality improvement process should be demonstrated as part of the systematic evaluation plan.

THE ACCREDITATION PROCESS

Accreditation relies upon a peer review process whereby evidence and standards are used to judge quality. Certain elements will always be present regardless of the agency conducting the accreditation process. Those elements focus on assessing the extent to which an institution or program meets a set of pre-established standards. Through the collection and analysis of data offered by the program, peers make a judgment (decision) regarding how successful the institution or program has been in demonstrating the achievement of the standards.

When the nursing program is ready to begin the accreditation process, programs would contact the selected accrediting agency, identify the types of programs seeking accreditation, and indicate the desire to start the formal steps of the accreditation process. The program will pay the accrediting agency a fee to cover the costs associated with the accreditation site visit and other aspects of the review process. The accrediting agency will provide the program with guidance on the typical timeline associated with the process. The program can then best determine when to plan for a program evaluation visit from the accrediting agency.

In the US, the accreditation process requires a series of steps designed to result in a comprehensive assessment and evaluation of program quality. The process allows the program to engage in a self-assessment of program strengths and areas for improvement and participate in the program's peer review of the program. The decision-making

---

BOX 5.4

Steps of the Accreditation Process

1. Engage in program assessment and processes that promote quality improvement.
2. Write a self-study report which offers an in-depth self-evaluation of performance associated with the agency standards of accreditation.
3. Host peer reviewers who conduct the program evaluation visit.
4. Render accrediting agency judgment (decision).
5. Monitor activities that verify the program continues to meet accreditor standards.
6. Re-evaluate to warrant continuation of accreditation.

Source: US Department of Education [USDE]. (2021). *Accreditation in the United States.* https://www2.ed.gov/admins/finaid/accred/accreditation_pg2.html

body for the accrediting agency will consider evidence from both the program's self-assessment and peer review process when rendering an accreditation decision. The steps usually associated with the accreditation process can be found in Box 5.4 and are discussed more fully in the following sections.

Ongoing Program Assessment

Many people may falsely believe that the accreditation process starts with a self-study; however, the journey to accreditation begins much earlier. The program needs to develop a systematic evaluation plan that provides a listing of the areas of evaluation, the person or group responsible for collecting data, the method or approach to the data collection, and the timing of the data collection. Once data has been collected, faculty need to analyze the results and determine appropriate actions. This ongoing assessment and analysis are part of the quality improvement process. On reviewing the collected data, faculty may determine that no changes are needed and continue their work, or changes may need to be initiated. Faculty will then want to continue to monitor these changes to determine effectiveness.

Self-Study: Program Self-Assessment

The accreditation process always begins with the program administrators, faculty, and staff conducting a self-assessment of how they perceive the program to be meeting the accrediting agency's accreditation standards. Conducting this review requires a thorough examination of a program's operations and performance in meeting the standards. Conducting such a process can take several months to complete, so the program must plan accordingly and develop a timeline that allows enough time for the self-assessment to be completed in a reflective, thorough, and comprehensive manner. This self-assessment phase of the accreditation process leads to a written narrative report that is commonly referred to as self-study. The self-study document, a detailed written report, addresses each accreditation standard and its criteria, providing data (evidence) of how the program meets the standard. In addition to the written narrative, documents that provide evidence of how the program meets the standards are also typically included in the report's appendices or shared as resources during the site visit. The self-study report shows how the program meets or exceeds the accreditation standards and provides an improvement plan as needed.

Each accrediting agency has policies and procedures regarding the self-study format. The writers of the self-study should carefully follow the accrediting agency's preparation and submission guidelines. The length of the self-study will vary depending on the number of programs being addressed within the document. The self-study document is typically submitted to the accrediting agency six to eight weeks before the scheduled program evaluation visit.

Peer Review: Program Evaluation Visit

Following submission of the program's self-study document, the program undergoes a site evaluation visit by a team of peer evaluators. Peer evaluators are volunteers and are not compensated for their services. The accrediting agency is responsible for appointing a team of evaluators, consisting of faculty and administrators from academia and nurses from practice. While the size of the team depends on the number of programs to be reviewed during the visit, it is most common to have a team of three or four program evaluators who complete the site visit over approximately three days. Complex programs with multiple sites or degree levels may require additional visitors or onsite review time. During the COVID-19 pandemic, accreditors have temporary flexibility regarding site visits, and they are allowed to conduct virtual site visits rather than in-person on-site visits. However, the USDE requires that a follow-up in-person focused visit must also occur to allow for on-site inspection when it is safe to do so (USDE, n.d.).

Regardless of the format of the visit, it is the responsibility of the program evaluation team to validate the data reported in the program's self-study document and seek any additional data needed to render a decision about the program's accreditation status. While conducting the visit for the nursing program, the evaluating team reviews additional program documents and interviews a variety of stakeholders, such as faculty, institutional and program administrators, students, employers, and alumni. The site evaluators also visit clinical sites and observe students and faculty in the classroom and clinical learning environment.

At the conclusion of the visit, the site visit team conducts an exit interview with the program, summarizing the team's findings regarding the program's compliance with each of the accreditation standards. It is not the responsibility of the site visit team to formulate any recommendations regarding the program's accreditation status; accreditation decisions are the sole responsibility of the accrediting agency's decision-making body, typically called a commission. Following the site visit, the evaluation team writes a report that outlines the team's findings and then submits the report to the accrediting agency. In turn, the accrediting agency provides a copy of the team report to the nursing program for review and response before forwarding the team report to the agency's accreditation review committee. The nursing program is given the opportunity to correct any *factual data* errors that may be contained in the report. Following the program's review and opportunity to respond, as appropriate, the next step in the accreditation process is for the program's self-study and site evaluation team report to be forwarded to the accrediting agency's review committee. Chapter 7 provides specific guidelines and helpful tips in preparing for the accreditation process.

Accrediting Agency Judgment (Decision)

The next step in the accreditation process involves rendering a decision regarding the program's accreditation status. The self-study document and the site evaluation team's written report form the basis for the accreditation decision. While the process may differ depending on the agency, it remains a peer review process. A common approach among nursing accrediting agencies is to forward the documentation to a review committee consisting of nurse educators and practice partners for consideration and to recommend a decision that is sent to the agency's board of commissioners for final action. Rendering the final accreditation decision is the responsibility of the agency's board, which is primarily composed of peers from education and practice and public members.

The decisions that are usually rendered fall into one of three categories:

1. Award accreditation of the program.
2. Accreditation of the program with conditions and a progress report required.
3. Accreditation denied.

In addition to the accreditation decision, the term of the accreditation is also granted. A program receiving initial accreditation will receive a shorter span of accreditation than programs being granted continuing accreditation. Depending on the nursing accrediting agency, an initial accreditation period is usually granted for five to six years. For programs seeking a continuation of their accreditation status, an accreditation term of up to a maximum of eight years (ACEN) or 10 years (CCNE and CNEA) may be granted. Table 5.2 compares the accreditation activities of the nursing accrediting agencies.

All accreditation decisions are a matter of public record. The accreditation agency is required to publicly disseminate the outcomes of their review process and send notice to the USDE. Programs are also required to publicly disclose the review's outcomes, and these are typically posted on the agency website (Hegji, 2020).

Monitoring Activities

After achieving initial accreditation, the program enters a continuing accreditation review cycle at designated times. Continuing accreditation usually requires the preparation of an updated self-study and another site evaluation visit. In between scheduled continuing accreditation visits, the program is required to pay annual fees and periodically send reports to the accrediting agency for review.

Accredited programs must submit required reports to the accreditation agency annually. Such reports capture data related to student outcomes, such as National Council Licensure Examination and certification pass rates; enrollment data; faculty numbers and qualifications; substantive changes in the program curricula, leadership, or financial status; and any other data the accrediting agency deems important to ongoing monitoring of the program. Accrediting agencies evaluate the data and determine if any concerning changes in the program may require a targeted visit to the program to gather additional information.

It is common for accrediting agencies to require a more extensive mid-cycle report from programs. They are asked to briefly address the accreditation standards and any changes that may have occurred since the last accreditation self-study and site visit. Through this reporting process, the program remains engaged in the continuous quality

TABLE 5.2

Comparison of Accreditation Activities for ACEN, CCNE, and CNEA

	ACEN	CCNE	CNEA
Candidacy period	Up to 2 years to host initial accreditation visit after notification of achieving candidacy	Must complete self-study and host an on-site evaluation within 2 years of date of acceptance as a new applicant Must have students enrolled for the equivalent of one academic year prior to hosting an on-site evaluation	Maximum of 3 years to complete the accreditation process
Maximum period of initial accreditation	5 years	5 years	6 years
Maximum period for continuing accreditation	8 years	10 years	10 years
Ongoing reporting/ monitoring	Yearly reports	Annual reports, compliance, and special reports as requested, Midterm continuous improvement progress report	Yearly reports and mid-cycle report
Notification of substantive changes such as administrator changes, curricular changes, or other changes	Required	Required	Required

Note: ACEN, Accreditation Commission for Education in Nursing; CCNE, Commission on Collegiate Nursing Education; CNEA, Commission for Nursing Education Accreditation.

Source: ACEN. (2020b). *Frequently asked questions.* https://www.acenursing.org/faq/; CCNE. (2021). *Procedures for accreditation of baccalaureate and graduate nursing programs.* https://www.aacnnursing.org/Portals/42/CCNE/PDF/Procedures.pdf; CNEA. (2019). *Accreditation handbook: Policies and procedures.* https://cnea.nln.org/resources

improvement process, and the accrediting agency is engaged in the ongoing review of the program's outcomes.

Re-evaluation

Since programs can change over time, accreditation is not indefinite. Nursing programs will need to be re-assessed and re-evaluated to determine if standards continue to be met. The time frame for this re-evaluation varies based upon the accrediting agency, but continuing accreditation occurs approximately every eight to 10 years. The program will continue with the assessment cycle and engage in another self-study and site visit as specified by the accrediting agency.

Summary

Accreditation plays a significant role in shaping US higher education. Engaging in a nursing accreditation review helps ensure quality improvement activities occur, and it also provides stakeholders with an assurance regarding program quality. Similarly, accreditation significantly impacts the quality and outcomes achieved in nursing education. By embracing accreditation as a contributor to systematic program evaluation and using the outcomes of the process to engage in program improvement, nursing faculty are accepting responsibility for providing students with quality education.

References

Accreditation Commission for Education in Nursing (ACEN). (2020a). *Accreditation manual: Section III: Standards and criteria.* https://www.acenursing.org/Resources-for-Nursing-Programs/sc2017-B.pdf

Accreditation Commission for Education in Nursing (ACEN). (2020b). *Frequently asked questions.* https://www.acenursing.org/faq/

Commission on Collegiate Nursing Education (CCNE). (2018a). *CCNE's 20th anniversary: 1998–2018.* https://www.aacnnursing.org/CCNE-Accreditation/20th-Anniversary

Commission on Collegiate Nursing Education (CCNE). (2018b). *Standards for accreditation of baccalaureate and graduate nursing programs.* https://www.aacnnursing.org/Portals/42/CCNE/PDF/Standards-Final-2018.pdf

Commission on Collegiate Nursing Education (CCNE). (2021). *Procedures for accreditation of baccalaureate and graduate nursing programs.* https://www.aacnnursing.org/Portals/42/CCNE/PDF/Procedures.pdf

Commission for Nursing Education Accreditation (CNEA). (2019). *Accreditation handbook: Policies and procedures.* https://cnea.nln.org/resources

Commission for Nursing Education Accreditation (CNEA). (2021). *Accreditation standards for nursing education programs.* https://cnea.nln.org/standards-of-accreditation

Hegji, A. (2020). *An overview of accreditation of higher education in the United States.* Congressional Research Service. https://sgp.fas.org/crs/misc/R43826.pdf

Kremer, M. J., & Horton, B. J. (2020). The accreditation process. In D. M. Billings & J. A. Halstead (Eds.), *Teaching in nursing: A guide for faculty* (6th ed., pp. 560–577). Elsevier.

National Council of State Boards of Nursing. (2020). A global profile of nursing regulation, education, and practice. *The Journal of Nursing Regulation, 10*(4), 1–112. https://www.ncsbn.org/14401.htm

National Council of State Boards of Nursing. (2021a). *Approval of nursing education programs.* https://www.ncsbn.org/665.htm

National Council of State Boards of Nursing. (2021b). *Guiding principles.* https://www.ncsbn.org/1325.htm

National League for Nursing. (2021). *History of the National League for Nursing 1893–2018.* http://www.nln.org/docs/default-source/default-document-library/nln-timeline-june-2020.pdf?sfvrsn=2

U.S. Department of Education. (n.d.). *Accreditation: Postsecondary institutions.* https://www.ed.gov/accreditation

U.S. Department of Education. (2021). *Accreditation in the United States.* https://www2.ed.gov/admins/finaid/accred/accreditation_pg12.html

U.S. Department of Education Office of Postsecondary Education Accreditation Group. (2020). *Accreditation handbook in accordance with 34 CFR Part 602 the secretary's recognition of accrediting agencies.* U.S. Department of Education. https://www2.ed.gov/admins/finaid/accred/accreditation-handbook.pdf

6

Developing a Systematic Program Evaluation Plan for a School of Nursing

Lynne Porter Lewallen, PhD, RN, CNE, ANEF

Nurse educators evaluate every day. An educator in the classroom or clinical area expects to evaluate students as part of this work. Nurse educators routinely do self-evaluations and peer evaluations, and administrators evaluate faculty and staff. But for some reason when it comes to program evaluation, the whole process can seem foreign. Systematic program evaluation (SPE) is critical for program improvement, as well as adherence to regulatory and accreditation standards. This chapter discusses the rationale for SPE and how to get started in creating a program evaluation plan or revising an existing plan. Areas to include in a plan are described, and samples of evaluation plan criteria using accreditation standards are provided.

WHY USE A PROGRAM EVALUATION PLAN?

With the many day-to-day expectations of a nurse educator, developing and using a program evaluation plan can seem like a low priority. It is easy to focus on one's own piece of the educational program, such as a single course or a certain level of student. This is important, but to truly assess the effectiveness of the program, a larger lens is required. A program evaluation plan helps faculty, administrators, and other stakeholders view the program as a whole and look at data over time to identify both positive and negative trends. This can provide a rationale for program changes or maintenance based on actual data. Additionally, the hallmark of evidence-based teaching is that new strategies are employed for individual courses or perhaps for entire programs. A program evaluation process can help faculty and administrators determine if these new strategies are successful (Royse et al., 2016).

REGULATORY AND ACCREDITATION INFLUENCES IN PROGRAM EVALUATION

Regulatory and accrediting bodies often require a written SPE, along with evidence of its use for program decision-making (Nunn-Ellison et al., 2018; Spector et al., 2018). Nursing has many regulatory and accreditation influences, and these are important to consider as the program develops a SPE plan. However, it is important to remember that the SPE belongs to the nursing program and needs to be useful in improving the particular program. If the plan is not useful, it will not be appropriate for accrediting and regulatory needs. If the faculty value the plan and see its usefulness, they will be more likely to implement it and make changes based on the data collected. There are several regulatory and accreditation factors to consider when developing and using a SPE plan.

Institutional Accrediting Bodies

Most nursing programs in the United States (US) are located within parent institutions that are accredited by one of the federally recognized institutional accrediting agencies (US Department of Education, 2021). Accrediting bodies such as the Southern Association of Colleges and Schools Commission on Colleges accredit the parent institution, which means the university, college, or community college in which the nursing program is located, enabling students to receive federal financial aid and transfer credits earned at the parent institution to other schools. These accreditors require that the parent institution collect and use evaluation data, such as student complaints, from each of its programs. The nursing program, and other units within the parent institution, collect and report data to the parent institution as a whole.

Although institutional accrediting bodies do not focus on individual programs and units within the institution, they require that the institution as a whole conducts program evaluation activities that examine the effectiveness and achievement of general college requirements and individual program outcomes. The nursing program is often required to participate in institution-wide quality enhancement plans (Southern Association of Colleges and Schools Commission on Colleges, n.d.). These plans identify key issues from the institution's own assessment plan to improve student learning outcomes and should be reflected in the SPE in the school of nursing.

Nursing Accrediting Bodies

Nursing accreditation standards are important to consider when developing a program evaluation plan. The accrediting bodies for nursing education that are approved by the U.S. Department of Education include the Accreditation Commission for Education in Nursing (ACEN, 2020); Commission on Collegiate Nursing Education (CCNE, 2018); and National League for Nursing Commission for Nursing Education Accreditation (CNEA) (National League for Nursing [NLN], 2021). These are programmatic accreditors. For nurse anesthesia programs, operating as stand-alone entities or within a larger nursing school or college, the Council on Accreditation of Nurse Anesthesia Educational Programs (COA) (COA, 2021) should also be considered. All these accrediting bodies have standards related to program outcomes. Specific required outcome measures vary, but all require evaluation of areas such as student learning outcomes, competencies of program graduates, and satisfaction of the employers of program graduates. The accrediting agencies require certain data to be collected, which would be reflected in the evaluation plan, and also require evidence that the data are used for program improvement. Accreditation is described further in Chapter 5.

State Boards of Nursing

Another agency affecting the evaluation of nursing programs is the state board of nursing. Approval of nursing programs by the state board is required in all states, although the criteria and processes vary. Some state boards of nursing require that nursing programs are accredited by national nursing accrediting bodies, but most do not (National Council of State Boards of Nursing [NCSBN], 2021). However, all state boards require evidence of program evaluation. Board of nursing requirements are often similar to those of nursing accrediting agencies but also may contain other specific requirements (Spector et al., 2018), all of which should be included in the SPE plan.

SUMMATIVE AND FORMATIVE EVALUATION

Program evaluation includes both summative and formative components. Summative (conclusive) evaluation is an assessment of the completed program (Royse et al., 2016; Stufflebeam & Zhang, 2017). For example, summative evaluation confirms whether the graduates of the program are prepared to enter the workforce for the role for which they were educated. With summative evaluation, the program is evaluating its product. Questions asked in the summative evaluation of a nursing program might include: Did we prepare our graduates to enter the workforce? Were our students able to achieve the end-of-program outcomes? Was the program efficient in terms of time, personnel, and cost? Are our stakeholders (graduates, alumni, employers) satisfied with graduates' performance? Common areas measured with summative evaluation include end-of-program student satisfaction and licensing/certification examination results.

Formative (process) evaluation of a nursing program occurs during the development and implementation of the program and its components (Royse et al., 2016; Stufflebeam & Zhang, 2017). Formative evaluation is an opportunity to collect data to make changes before the program is completed. This type of evaluation can help determine if the best outcomes are being produced with the least expense in terms of time, effort, stress, finances, and use of resources. This is a detailed evaluation, which includes the evaluation of processes. With formative evaluation, changes can be made immediately. Questions asked in formative evaluation might include: Is the content being delivered as planned — does the plan have fidelity? Are the students progressing through the earlier courses in the curriculum? Are the chosen clinical sites able to provide the students with appropriate experiences to achieve the course learning outcomes? Formative evaluation allows for revision of courses and other changes in the program. Common areas measured with formative evaluation include results of achievement tests early in the nursing program, reports of adequacy and availability of clinical sites, and student satisfaction surveys administered at the end of or during courses.

DEVELOPING A SYSTEMATIC PROGRAM EVALUATION PLAN

When beginning to develop a SPE plan, it is important to decide on criteria for evaluation to include in it. An organizing framework can help with this decision. Some programs organize their SPE plans by accreditation or approval criteria; however, with this approach, the program also may want to evaluate additional areas not included in the criteria that are nevertheless important to the program. The sample evaluation criteria included in this chapter are based on nursing accreditation standards.

Other nursing programs prefer to use an evaluation model to organize the SPE plan. Although evaluation models can be useful, most are not designed for nursing programs specifically, so care must be taken to also include all the areas required for regulatory and accrediting consideration. There are numerous evaluation models in the literature from which to choose; a popular one is the CIPP (Context, Input, Process, Product) model (Stufflebeam & Zhang, 2017). The CIPP model, introduced in Chapter 1, examines intended ends and means as compared to actual ends and means. The four major areas of evaluation with this model are: (1) context (intended ends), (2) input (intended means), (3) process (actual means), and (4) product (actual ends). This model could be used to design an overall program evaluation plan or to assess a specific area of concern in the nursing program.

For context, what the program intends to accomplish, some areas of evaluation would include the needs of both internal and external stakeholders, and the setting in which the program is situated. Nurse educators should ask: What are the expectations of employers of the graduates? In what types of settings is employment available? Where do students in our program come from, and where do the graduates typically go? What type of parent institution houses the nursing program, and what type of program fits within the mission of the institution? In the area of input, which considers whether the program design and resources accomplish program goals, areas of evaluation would include faculty and staff adequacy to conduct the nursing program; physical, online, and clinical resources; support for online education; university and nursing support for students; adequacy of prerequisite courses outside the nursing discipline, if applicable for the program; and the budgetary resources necessary to fund program needs. For process, considering how the program design is actually working, evaluation areas would focus on the ability to schedule adequate amounts of appropriate clinical experiences; if the curriculum met all applicable professional standards; if resources such as tutoring were sufficient to meet actual needs; and if the planned content is able to be covered in the courses as designed. In the area of product, measuring how the actual program outcomes compare to the intended outcomes, some areas of evaluation would be if graduates are able to meet the end-of-program outcomes and pass licensure and certification examinations if the graduates are able to obtain appropriate employment, and if employers are satisfied with graduates' performance.

COMPONENTS OF A SYSTEMATIC PROGRAM EVALUATION PLAN

Once the evaluation criteria have been established, the plan should be structured to facilitate data gathering, analysis, and use for program improvement. The sample criteria in this chapter use a table format as a structure, which is a common method. The table can be customizable to the nursing program but at a minimum should include the area of evaluation (commonly referred to as the criterion), expected level of achievement (ELA), person or group responsible for collecting the data, method of assessment of the criterion, and timeframe in which the data are collected (Box 6.1). Most SPE plans also include columns to record the actual data collected and actions taken resulting from analysis of those data. Generally, the plan covers one academic year.

> **BOX 6.1**
>
> ### Areas to Include in Program Evaluation Document
>
> The following areas should be included in your systematic program evaluation document:
>
> Criterion (area of evaluation)
> Expected level of achievement
> Person or group responsible for collecting the data
> Method of assessment
> Timeframe
> Actual data collected
> Actions taken

Areas of Evaluation

The areas of evaluation should encompass applicable accreditation requirements but also may contain other areas of importance to the school of nursing. For example, a nursing program may evaluate the cost-effectiveness of offering all or part of a course online. Nursing programs often have not had processes in place to conduct cost-benefit analyses, but the costs of higher education have become an issue for consumers, funders, and institutions themselves (Gordon, 2018). This is an area to consider adding to a SPE plan. Areas of evaluation to include in the plan are discussed further in the next section of the chapter.

Expected Level of Achievement (ELA)

The ELA for each criterion should be developed thoughtfully. Sometimes the ELA is prescribed by an external body. For example, the CNEA requires that the three-year average of the first-time pass rate on the National Council Licensure Examination (NCLEX) be at least 80% (NLN, 2021), whereas ACEN requires that the first-time NCLEX pass rate be at least 80% for each calendar year (ACEN, 2020). CCNE (2018) allows either of these standards to be used. In this case, the program must meet a particular standard to remain in compliance with the accrediting agency. For other criteria, such as faculty scholarship, the program may be able to set its own benchmarks. This is illustrated in CCNE's requirement that the program set faculty outcomes that are appropriate to the institution's mission and expectations (CCNE, 2018). It is important to set benchmarks that are reasonable for the nursing program based on factors such as past performance. While it may be tempting to set high goals, which the program is not likely to meet, the program may then be continually in an area of deficit, explaining benchmarks were not met.

A better plan is to establish a reasonable benchmark, with a long-term goal to increase it. Using faculty scholarship as an example, a long-term goal might be for each tenure-track faculty member to publish two articles in peer-reviewed journals per year. If the current baseline average is 0.5 articles per year, two for the next year is not a reasonable goal. Therefore, the first-year benchmark might be one per year, with the addition of an organized writing group for faculty to accomplish this goal. At the end of the year, evaluation data can lead the program to either increase the benchmark, if the goal was met, or improve the support systems for faculty if the goal was not met.

Responsible Person or Groups

The individuals or groups responsible for collecting the data should be identified for each criterion. It is important that this be specific: a general group such as "all faculty" may not result in data being collected systematically. Some larger schools of nursing may have a specific person or office that collects all of the evaluation data; in smaller schools, the program director may have the primary responsibility. Ultimately, however, evaluation is more successful if the responsibility to collect data is shared among the faculty and administrators. This responsibility should be clearly defined with a mechanism for reporting the data. For example, if the curriculum committee is responsible for collecting data on the percentage of simulation in each clinical course, the Chair might have an annual report requirement with this as a clearly identified question to answer. Although one person or group may be responsible for the overall final audit of the SPE plan, including others in the data gathering and aggregation increases awareness of the importance of program evaluation and can lead to more useful measures being employed (Danley-Scott & Scott, 2017).

Another structure that can be used for collecting evaluation data is current committees in the school. For example, the curriculum committee might be responsible for collecting course evaluations, and a student affairs committee might be responsible for collecting student satisfaction data.

Method of Assessment

Another consideration is the method of assessment of each criterion. For example, if the program has a criterion for graduate satisfaction, then the instrument used to collect this information should have a question or a scale that specifically measures satisfaction. While this sounds self-evident, it is not uncommon for evaluation instruments to be designed in isolation from the criteria they are intended to measure. Additionally, some areas that are important to measure are complex, such as the student's ability to meet all the program outcomes. An important point to remember is that there are many ways to evaluate whether the program is meeting the criteria in the SPE plan. It is not necessary to collect data using all possible evaluation methods; typically, one or two will suffice.

Timeframe

The evaluation plan should include a specified timeframe in which the data are collected, such as at the end of each semester or academic year. By setting a specific timeframe, it is easier to determine when to aggregate the data for reporting and action purposes.

Results

Many SPE plans also include a column for actual results. In that column, the data related to each criterion can be recorded for that academic year including the source of the data, such as the minutes of a particular meeting, which allows auditors to track the data and confirm the results. The program must have adequate documentation of both the data and decisions made. Minutes of meetings should have details about the discussions of aggregated outcomes and decisions based on those discussions. Decisions should be followed up, with this process also documented. The discussions can be labeled in the meeting minutes with the evaluation plan criterion number, not only making it easy to track these discussions but also having the added benefit of keeping faculty aware of the SPE. For areas that are evaluated regularly, schools can set a certain time a year for aggregating the data and reporting the results to stakeholders. It is critical that results of program evaluation are actually used for decision-making, not merely reported. All faculty, both full- and part-time, should have input into decisions based on data (Danley-Scott & Scott, 2017).

Actions Taken

The final column on the plan may contain the actions taken based on the evaluation. These actions should be specific, allowing for follow-up during the next year. For example, the pass rates of an advanced practice certification exam may be trending downward over three years. The action may be to contact the director and faculty of the APRN program to ask for a discussion of this trend and a plan to reverse it. A specific plan like this provides adequate information for follow-up on this criterion and the exam pass rates for the next year. This column also can include plans for change, which should be specific to allow tracking the process of change during the next academic year. If the data show that the criterion is being met, this column may indicate simply maintenance of the current process.

STRUCTURE OF PROGRAM EVALUATION PLAN

Although the program evaluation plan should be tailored to the specific program, the structure of the plans can look similar in different programs. In this section of the chapter, examples are provided of evaluation plans that illustrate the process and each of the components of evaluation. The samples use criteria from each of the three major programmatic accreditation agencies. It is often useful to have one document that contains the entire SPE plan. If the school of nursing offers multiple nursing programs, separate sections can focus on a particular program. However, having one document can ensure nothing is missed.

Whether the program uses accreditation standards or an evaluation model to guide the structure of the evaluation plan, there are certain areas that all programs need to evaluate. Depending on the model or accreditation standards on which the SPE is based, these areas may have different names and be organized differently. For clarity, they will be described here separately under the headings of administration, faculty, students, curriculum, resources (including cost and efficiency), and program outcomes.

Administration

The area of administration is concerned with how the nursing program and the larger parent institution fit and work together. Nursing programs should be able to demonstrate how their program fits within the mission of the parent institution. This is often demonstrated with tables comparing the mission and vision of the parent institution with the mission, vision, and goals of the nursing program. If either the nursing program or parent institution revises the mission or goals, congruence between them should be reassessed, and the need for additional revision to assure congruence should be discussed. Documentation of faculty, student, and other community of interest members' participation in the work of the institution and nursing program is necessary and is often accomplished with a list of committee assignments and records of attendance.

When students are part of committees, it is important to document their attendance in the minutes and note instances in which student input was used, even if the students were not present at the meeting. One way this can be accomplished is by discussing student feedback, formal or informal, about an issue and deciding on a course of action as a result of that feedback. In one medical school, a student representative for each class was appointed to poll students for their feedback regarding the clinical placement process, resulting in student satisfaction and helpful information for faculty planning the placements (Russel et al., 2021). Documentation of how students are informed of the results of evaluation of the data would close the loop.

An additional area to consider is the integrity, or accuracy, of public information about the nursing program. This involves clear communication about areas such as the admission and progression policies, grievance procedures, course offerings, and program plans. Public information can exist in many platforms, such as websites, catalogs, brochures, handbooks, and recruitment materials. One person could be assigned to monitor the consistency of information across these many venues. It would also be important to note information and links about the nursing program that may be housed within different departments of the parent institution, to make sure that information remains accurate. The integrity of public information should be assessed at least annually. Table A.1 in Appendix A provides an example of a completed evaluation plan for faculty and student participation in program governance.

Faculty

The area of faculty can incorporate qualifications, support, work assignments, and program-specific expectations. Data collected related to faculty who teach in the nursing program may include degrees held, progress toward advanced degrees, licensure, certifications, maintenance of clinical expertise, and continuing education. The goal is to document how faculty remain qualified for their positions. Qualifications of preceptors usually are described in this category as well. The amount of data about faculty can be difficult to aggregate in a way that is useful for the program. For this reason, it is helpful to identify a few key areas to evaluate and develop processes to make those data available for aggregation. Two areas that outside stakeholders often monitor closely are the degrees and licensure/certifications of faculty and the amount and type of continuing education faculty members complete. Generally, degrees, licensure and certification, and continuing education program attended can be listed easily, but more challenging can be the decision about whether the continuing education enabled faculty members to maintain their expertise. Aggregate, program-wide goals for faculty development or performance are often monitored by accrediting agencies and may have a specific focus, such as continuing education related to teaching (COA, 2021) or be determined by the program (ACEN, 2020; CCNE, 2018; NLN, 2021).

Many nursing programs have position descriptions and guidelines for promotion and tenure or similar guidelines for faculty not on tenure-track that specify the expectations of faculty. If the data show that faculty members are not consistently meeting position expectations, areas to consider in the program evaluation might be if workloads are too high or if there are insufficient faculty development opportunities. This is a good illustration of how categories of evaluation are not mutually exclusive. An excessive workload may indicate a problem with administrative support to hire additional nurse educators; a deficit in faculty development could indicate inadequate resources for professional development, a lack of time for faculty to attend continuing education, or a lack of offerings in the area. Table A.2 in Appendix A provides an example of a completed evaluation plan to assess faculty expertise.

Students

Students are the reason nursing programs exist, and programs should evaluate not only student progress to a degree (usually measured under the outcomes area) but also services available to students and the student experience of the educational process. Areas to evaluate concerning students are the availability of student services including services for students who learn online or at distant sites, maintenance of student records including financial aid records, and clear explanation of student policies. Financial aid information is often monitored by the parent institution if it is institutionally accredited, but for stand-alone nursing programs, this is an important area to document. Some nursing accrediting agencies, such as the ACEN and COA, serve as gatekeepers for federal financial aid assessment. Formative evaluation is especially important in the area of students. There should be mechanisms in place for students to express concerns quickly to resolve small problems before they escalate. Programs also should evaluate how student complaints are handled to make sure students receive due process. This is a requirement of institutional and nursing accrediting bodies, and parent institutions frequently monitor this process for each unit within the institution. Table A.3 in Appendix A is an example of an assessment of the student complaints process.

Curriculum

The curriculum is the heart of the nursing program and making sure the curriculum is functioning to facilitate program outcomes is a primary aspect of program evaluation. Important areas to include in a SPE plan related to the curriculum are an assessment of how the curriculum incorporates professional standards and practice realities, how each course is evaluated and the relationship of that process to the evaluation of the overall curriculum, and how clinical sites contribute to students' ability to meet course and program student learning outcomes. Data to monitor include the minutes of course and curriculum committee meetings, clinical site evaluation forms, students' performance on standardized tests as a reflection of how the curriculum meets national norms, employers' satisfaction with graduates as a reflection of how the curriculum addresses practice realities, and student and faculty evaluation of courses for both formative and summative purposes. It is critical to retain minutes of all meetings at which curriculum matters are discussed— these provide documentation for the evaluation plan and a record of decisions about the curriculum. Accrediting bodies require that faculty members be involved in the development, evaluation, and revision of the curriculum, and this is an area in which documentation is frequently lacking. Table A.4 in Appendix A provides an example of assessment of faculty participation in curriculum development, evaluation, and revision.

Resources

Resources vary tremendously among programs, but all programs need resources to function. The category of resources is broad and includes all the human, physical, learning, and fiscal resources that affect the nursing program. This is an area that is often neglected in an SPE because resources may not have a natural end point for measurements, such as the end of a program or an academic year. Human resources to be assessed include the adequacy of both faculty and staff, such as academic advisors, information technology (IT) support, and clerical personnel. Examples of records to maintain include the number of student visits to advisors, number of consultations for IT support and typical wait time for both faculty and students, and typical lead time required for faculty members to receive clerical support. Additional data to collect include budgetary support of the nursing program, both in comparison with other comparable programs in the institution and in relation to the work of the nursing program, for example, funding for adequate numbers of faculty. Physical resource assessment includes areas such as classroom size and technology adequacy, faculty office adequacy, clinical site effectiveness in providing opportunities to practice necessary skills, and clinical laboratory and simulation opportunities. Technology availability and support have become increasingly critical with more students and faculty working remotely either full-time or sporadically. Learning resources can include the library, including online resources, online simulation programs, and the availability of tutoring. Fiscal resources include funding for faculty positions, salary increases, staff support, faculty development and travel, and equipment purchases. If the school of nursing offers programs at a distance, it is important to assess resources that contribute to both student and faculty success in this learning format. See Appendix A, Table A.5, for an example of an assessment of physical resources.

Program Outcomes

Program outcomes are commonly measured as part of a SPE and are required to be reported to most accrediting and regulatory bodies. Outcomes measurement relies heavily on external sources of information, such as surveys of employers, thus access to those sources is an important consideration. To effectively evaluate the overall achievement of program outcomes, they need to be well defined, and multiple measures should be used. Internal measures might include an assessment of a comprehensive project, such as a portfolio, capstone project, thesis, or dissertation. Examples of external measures are first-time pass rates on licensure and certification examinations, scores on comprehensive tests, and employer satisfaction with the graduates' performance. Programs should consider tracking both aggregated and strategically disaggregated outcomes data, which can provide insight into issues of equity and diversity (Jeffreys, 2021). For example, do students in a certain cohort progress more seamlessly through a program? Do students in certain demographic groups gain degree-related employment faster?

One type of data that is collected in this area is the length of time for students to complete the program. Accrediting agencies, boards of nursing, and parent institutions monitor program completion rates and may have specific benchmarks to which programs are held. This is an area where frequent recording of data is helpful. Accrediting agencies sometimes provide guidance on the calculation of program completion rates depending on why the student left the program (e.g., CCNE 2018, Standard IV-B), so keeping up with this information as students exit the program without graduating can assist with these calculations.

Data collected from graduates of the program include perceptions of their achievement of program outcomes; satisfaction with the program including courses, quality and responsiveness of the faculty, clinical experiences, learning resources, and the grievance and complaint process; and readiness to assume the role for which they were prepared. Typically, this information is collected near the end of the last semester of enrollment. If students have been offered a position prior to graduation, it is valuable to collect employment information before they leave, since contacting them as alumni may prove challenging.

Of the three major nursing accrediting bodies, CNEA (NLN, 2021) is the only one that requires collection of alumni data. Data collected from alumni include their achievement of program outcomes, their satisfaction with the program, information about the type of position they obtained and preparation for it, licensure and certifications, progression to advanced degrees, leadership roles, publications, and professional presentations, among others. Alumni information is collected typically at a time point between six months and one year after graduation, although some schools of nursing also collect data at later intervals.

Because nursing is a practice profession, it is critical that graduates contribute to the practice arena, and employers are in the best position to assess this ability. The employers of graduates of the program can provide important information about the graduates' ability to function in the position for which they were hired and the graduate's readiness for entry into practice. Other general information that can be gathered from employers includes new skills being required of graduates and areas in which they need extensive orientation; this type of information may be useful to the program in making decisions about curriculum revisions. Employers also should be consulted as new programs are considered for development.

Table A.6 in Appendix A provides an example of the assessment of graduates' employment. In this example, aggregated data are reported, which allows faculty to assess the program's achievement of the overall criterion. While the results in this example meet benchmarks, in some programs the response rate for the surveys is low, leading to concern about the usefulness of the data given the small sample size. The risk of a biased sample is high, and the program may not have enough data on which to base conclusions and revisions.

CHALLENGING AREAS TO EVALUATE: GATHERING OUTCOMES DATA FROM GRADUATES, ALUMNI, AND EMPLOYERS

Surveys are a common method of collecting data from graduates, alumni, and employers. They allow the program to collect specific data from a large number of respondents and do so quickly. However, low response rates for surveys are a common problem

(Carr et al., 2018). Electronic surveys are less costly and may yield a better response rate than mailed surveys because they are faster to complete; however, email addresses change frequently, and bounce-backs may be common. It is useful to obtain students' personal email addresses before they graduate from the program, even if the institution allows them to keep their student email addresses. This may facilitate contact later. If possible, programs might want to consider incentives for completing surveys. There has been concern about fraudulent survey results, however, especially for surveys where incentives are offered. In some cases, uninvited people or bots can gain access to online surveys and complete them to obtain the incentives, so the results of online surveys should be examined for suspicious results or response patterns (Levi et al., 2022).

Another way to collect data from graduates is through focus groups. Although focus groups include fewer people than would a survey, the program may obtain richer data for use in program evaluation. Focus groups could be held between the last day of class and graduation, when memories are fresh and grading is completed, or at times when orientation groups meet at the largest employers of graduates of the program. Social media also can be used to collect data about program outcomes and provide access to surveys. Many nurses are active on social media (Fredericks & Duong, 2020), and sites such as Facebook can be used to discover employment locations, seek comments about the nursing program, and include links to online surveys.

Many graduates keep in touch with one or two faculty members and may provide information about new positions, graduate school, and experiences that would be helpful for the program in considering improvements. If there were an established mechanism for faculty to easily document that information, it could be aggregated for program evaluation purposes.

In addition to contacting alumni by mail, email, or social media, they can be reached in other ways, especially if they tend to be concentrated in one geographic area. The nursing program can set up tables at major employers at lunchtime to talk to alumni; this strategy can be used to gather employment data, collect brief survey data, and recruit alumni for higher degree programs if offered by the school. This same strategy could be employed at nursing organization or community meetings; an alumni reception or table can facilitate the gathering of data. Events held by the parent institution, such as homecoming, also provide a place to make contact with alumni for program evaluation. If the parent institution has an alumni association, that group may be a source of alumni contact and employer information.

To collect data from employers, similar strategies can be used as described earlier for alumni. Frequently, employers will attend similar nursing conferences and community events as alumni and can be reached in the same way. Other strategies to reach employers are periodic focus groups for lunch and contact at regular meetings agency representatives attend, such as clinical coordination meetings. Most nursing programs have advisory boards, of which alumni and employers of graduates may be members; that group can provide valuable information and may suggest other contacts to facilitate gathering a wider sampling of data. It is also recommended to reach out to alumni who employ graduates of the program. Although it is not possible to contact every employer of every graduate, important data can be collected by speaking to smaller groups that are representative of the types of agencies that employ program graduates. During the

COVID pandemic, the use of electronic real-time meetings became common. Meeting electronically can be a continued way to meet with employers and may be more attractive than face-to-face meetings due to the elimination of travel time and parking issues common on college campuses. Many of these platforms allow creation of breakout rooms, which can be useful for focus group data collection in conjunction with larger group discussions. Videoconferencing has been shown to allow for productive interactivity in focus groups (Henage et al., 2021).

EVALUATE PROCESS

Finally, it is important to evaluate periodically the SPE plan. As faculty, administrators, and other stakeholders use the plan, they should identify areas in which the criteria need to be changed and measures that may not provide the needed data. As accreditation standards change, the plan will need revision. The program evaluation plan should be a "living document"—one that is used and amended as necessary to serve the program's purposes. Results of key measures should be communicated to stakeholders so they can provide input. This can be done in a variety of mechanisms, such as reports at meetings, information posted on websites, or electronic dashboards (Opsahl & Horton-Deutsh, 2019).

Program evaluation is critical to ensuring the success of the program, but it must be systematic and planned. If program evaluation can be integrated into the normal workflow of the program, it is less burdensome and will generate data for program improvement.

Summary

This chapter identified influences on program evaluation processes, both internal and external, in the institution in which the nursing program is housed. Common areas to be included in program evaluation plans were discussed, with sample criteria based on national nursing accrediting body standards. Finally, ideas for gathering data in challenging areas were presented.

References

Accreditation Commission for Education in Nursing. (2020). *Accreditation manual.* https://www.acenursing.org/acen-accreditation-manual/

Carr, D., Boyle, E. H., Cornwell, B., Correll, S., Crosnoe, R., Freese, J., & Waters, M. C. (2018). *The art and science of social research.* W.W. Norton.

Commission on Collegiate Education in Nursing. (2018). *Standards for accreditation of baccalaureate and graduate degree nursing programs.* https://www.aacnnursing.org/Portals/42/CCNE/PDF/Standards-Final-2018.pdf

Council on Accreditation of Nurse Anesthesia Educational Programs [COA]. (2021). *Accreditation standards, policies and procedures, and guidelines.* https://www.coacrna.org/accreditation/accreditation-standards-policies-and-procedures-and-guidelines/

Danley-Scott, J., & Scott, G. (2017). Why all faculty should have a seat at the assessment table. *Journal of Assessment and Institutional*

Effectiveness, 7(1–2), 20–40. https://muse.jhu.edu/article/711007

Fredericks, S., & Duong, J. (2020). Using social media to network, converse, and build community within graduate nursing education. *Canadian Journal of Nursing Informatics, 24*(3). Retrieved June 12, 2022, from https://cjni.net/journal/?p=5864

Gordon, G. (2018). The cost-effectiveness of public higher education: Integrating accounting and quality to assess value. *Journal of Accounting and Finance, 18*(10), 19–30. doi:10.33423/JAF.V18I10.231

Henage, C. B., Ferreri, S. P., Schlusser, C., Hughes, T. D., Armistead, L. T., Kelley, C. J., Niznik, J. D., Busby-Whitehead, J., & Roberts, E. (2021). Transitioning focus group research to a videoconferencing environment: A descriptive analysis of interactivity. *Pharmacy, 9*(3), 117. doi:10.3390/pharmacy9030117

Jeffreys, M. R. (2021). Data analytics in nursing education: Trended tracking matters for theory, research, and practice. *Teaching and Learning in Nursing, 16*, 181–188. https://doi.org/10.1016/j.teln.2021.01.003

Levi, R., Ridberg, R., Akers, M., & Seligman, H. (2022). Survey fraud and the integrity of web-based survey research. *American Journal of Health Promotion, 36*(1), 18–20. doi:10.1177/08901171211037531

National Council of State Boards of Nursing. (2021). *Approval of nursing education programs.* https://www.ncsbn.org/665.htm

National League for Nursing. (2021). *NLN CNEA standards for accreditation.* https://cnea.nln.org/standards-of-accreditation

Nunn-Ellison, K., Ard, N., Beasley, S. F., & Farmer, S. (2018). Systematic plan of evaluation part II: Assessment of program outcomes. *Teaching and Learning in Nursing, 13*, 113–118. https://doi.org/10.1016/j.teln.2017.11.001

Opsahl, A., & Horton-Deutsch, S. (2019). A nursing dashboard to communicate the evaluation of program outcomes. *Nurse Educator, 44*(6), 326–329. doi: 10.1097/NNE.0000000000000632

Royse, D., Thyer, B., & Padgett, D. (2016). *Program evaluation: An introduction to an evidence-based approach* (6th ed.). Delmar Cengage Learning.

Russel, S. M., Geraghty, J. R., Kobayashi, K. R., Patel, S., Stringham, R., Hyderi, A., & Curry, R. H. (2021). Evaluating core clerkships: Lessons learned from implementing a student-driven feedback system for clinical curricula. *Academic Medicine, 96*(2), 232–235. doi: 10.1097/ACM.0000000000003760

Southern Association of Colleges and Schools Commission on Colleges. (n.d.). The quality enhancement plan. https://sacscoc.org/app/uploads/2020/01/Quality-Enhancement-Plan-1.pdf

Spector, N., Hooper, J. I., Silvestre, J., & Qian, H. (2018). Board of nursing approval of registered nurse education programs. *Journal of Nursing Regulation, 8*(4), 18–31.

Stufflebeam, D. L., & Zhang, G. (2017). *The CIPP evaluation model: How to evaluate for improvement and accountability.* The Guilford Press.

U.S. Department of Education. (2021). *Accreditation in the United States.* https://www2.ed.gov/admins/finaid/accred/accreditation.html#Overview

7

Program Evaluation: Getting It Done in Your School of Nursing

Diana M. Vergara, MA
John M. Clochesy, PhD, MA, RN

Accreditation is a vital process whereby schools/colleges of nursing meet identified standards for the implementation and continuation of nursing programs at all levels. The review process for accreditation is rigorous and holds programs to the highest standards of nursing education. By successfully adhering to accreditation standards, schools of nursing can assure prospective students, graduates, and employers of the quality of their programs and may enable schools/colleges to seek federal financial aid for students. Preparing for accreditation can be overwhelming. In this chapter, the authors offer some specific guidelines and helpful tips for preparing for the accreditation process in your school of nursing.

WHO SHOULD BE INVOLVED

All members of the school of nursing community should be involved in the accreditation process. This is an opportunity for faculty, students, and staff to showcase with pride their school through the preliminary accreditation writing processes, building the resource base, designing an accreditation team room, and interacting with the accreditation team when they arrive. The preparation process for an accreditation review should begin 18 to 24 months prior to the accreditation team site visit, whether it is in-person, virtual, or hybrid. The roles and responsibilities of faculty and staff need to be defined early in the process. Writing groups should be formed for each of the accreditation standards and their respective key elements. Faculty and staff participate in preparing the self-study, adhering to a strict timeline with predetermined deadlines. Ideally, these groups should be led by a facilitator with prior accreditation experience. To establish documentation standards and quality control, oversee deadlines, and ensure momentum is not lost over the extended time frame, a few select faculty and staff should be identified as the leaders of the project.

Our Process

In our school of nursing, the process began almost two years prior to the accreditation review and team site visit. Preparation for the accreditation review was treated as a large project, with several components: (1) the self-study report, (2) required documentation and data (the resource room), and (3) site visit preparation. A timeline was created to keep everyone on task, and deadlines were diligently adhered to and revised as needed. The editors of the final version of the self-study report, a faculty member and a staff member, served as the main point personnel for the accreditation "project." Writing groups ranged from six to 10 members each and were formed for each of the accreditation standards related to programs and respective key elements. Faculty voluntarily joined the standard writing groups based on general interest, prior curriculum planning, committee membership, or accreditation experience. This allowed faculty to be engaged with the information. Also, it was clear to all that faculty were part of the self-study process when they met with members of the site visit team. Depending on the accreditation standards, it is important that faculty and other members of the communities of interest be engaged in the self-study process.

Associate deans for the undergraduate and graduate programs served as facilitators, and both undergraduate and graduate faculty were included in each writing group. Staff were assigned to groups based on relevant experience and their roles in the school. For example, the National League for Nursing Commission for Nursing Education Accreditation (CNEA) Standard I, related to program outcomes, was facilitated largely by the editors as they were the school's central data custodians for information such as graduation and licensure rates (National League for Nursing, 2021). For the standard related to the mission, governance, and resources (CNEA Standard II), key staff, such as human resources and financial officers, were involved. Those writing for CNEA Standards III (faculty) and V (curriculum and evaluation) had the largest number of faculty and academic staff, as this standard dealt with faculty, curriculum, and teaching and learning processes. Program faculty and staff from the student services office participated in writing about students (CNEA Standard IV). Box 7.1 provides tips for assembling faculty and staff into groups to prepare the self-study.

BOX 7.1

Tips for Establishing Faculty and Staff Teams to Prepare Self-Study

- Choose facilitators who have prior experience with the accreditation process.
- Choose team members with the expertise required for each Standard.
- Create an 18- to 24-month timeline with specific deadlines.
- Preassign staff with responsibility for each step in the accreditation process.
- Preassign staff with responsibility for any required documentation.
- Present and share the timeline and schedule with all faculty and staff (if shared in a central location, everyone in the school can know the status of the accreditation process over time).
- Assign one person to be responsible for the timeline and notification to groups as to their deadlines approach.
- Assign data custodians for all documentation and data points for the report.
- Create an atmosphere of group pride and responsibility.
- Schedule recurring agenda items to update relevant committees and groups.

SETTING UP PROCESSES FOR ACCREDITATION

It is important to start the planning process at least 18 months prior to the accreditation site visit. Planning may include a visit to the accreditation headquarters or participation in conferences and workshops sponsored by the accrediting body to review successful accreditation reports and collect pertinent information to make the accreditation process progress smoothly. Often, reviewing the report from a school that recently underwent a successful accreditation visit may be helpful. Accreditation should be a standing agenda item at all appropriate committee meetings.

Our Process

When we started planning for accreditation, we discovered through the initial review that despite the copious collection of evaluation data over the years, there was not a systematic review process nor was there a central repository of all relevant data and documentation. From this point on, the Director of Evaluation in the dean's office was solely responsible for conducting, analyzing, and reporting evaluation data. The dean's office was now the central repository for all evaluation data. This was of great help for any external requests for information. Additionally, in our process, the editors were responsible for setting specific timelines for each standard to facilitate clear expectations for the standards' groups and other contributors to adhere to. Figure 7.1 provides a sample worksheet that programs can use to set timelines and track the progress of the accreditation project. We reviewed the accrediting body's website for templates and resources on how to format the report and appendices; this was not a one-day process as templates, and resources can change in the 18- to 24-month timespan.

The writing groups can begin to document the process of analyzing five-year trends and establishing new benchmarks, reviewing student satisfaction and alumni surveys related to outcomes, and examining data on student and employer satisfaction with the program—in essence, program effectiveness. The school governance structure and bylaws may reveal which committees have already done this internal evaluation process if it is not formalized through an evaluation committee. For instance, in our school, faculty regularly reviewed outcome data in curriculum committees and program director meetings. We collected copies of all such committee minutes through their shared central repository for submission to the writing groups to assist in writing the self-study.

Simultaneously, other processes were taking shape in preparing for the site visit. Accreditation became a standing agenda item in all faculty committee and school council meetings, and a recurring item at administrative staff meetings. At these meetings, faculty and staff were apprised of the purpose of the self-study and preparation process and presented with proposed deadlines for report preparation and the site visit. The editors developed and used visual timelines and project planning guides, as the majority of faculty and staff were not well versed in the breadth of accreditation requirements, and the large scale of self-study reports and site visits. Emphasis was on the importance of program effectiveness, outcomes, and how the self-study could help us bring about improvement relative to the changes we had initiated over

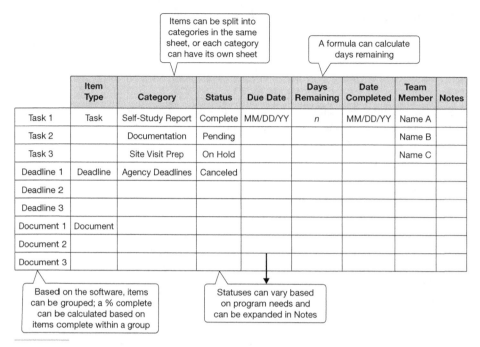

FIGURE 7.1 Sample project management worksheet.

the previous 10 years. The respective groups presented drafts on standard-specific progress to the authors and associate deans. Most questions raised were answered by the group facilitator. However, in cases of ambiguity, detailed notes were taken and clarification was sought through the official accreditation contact person at the accreditation office.

As the site visit became closer, meetings were held with select faculty (e.g., undergraduate faculty, graduate faculty, and committees). These were held with the purpose of reflecting on and answering questions about the accreditation report, such as:

1. Did the self-study report address the expectations set forth in each standard or key element?
2. Could the clarity of the draft report be enhanced by using tables?
3. What are strengths and areas for improvement with respect to the draft report?
4. What, if anything, is vague or unclear?

We notified colleagues at our clinical partners' organizations of the impending accreditation dates and details. The goal was to facilitate value and participation by all members of our community of interest. These members included the university and college administrators; external stakeholders (hospitals, nursing homes, the local technical college); and other schools of nursing within our region. Leaders from our partner organizations were invited to meet with the site visit evaluators as members of our community of interest.

Some strategies for setting up accreditation processes include:

> Visit websites to review accreditation report formatting.
> If possible, visit the accreditation headquarters to review successful accreditation reports and collect pertinent information to make the process go smoothly.
> Establish clearly defined roles and expectations for those involved in the accreditation process, including those who will serve as data/project managers and liaisons to the accrediting bodies.
> Contact clinical partners early to help them understand the accreditation process and obtain their support.
> At least 18 to 24 months in advance, review all required data points and documentation and, if needed, create a digital central repository.
> Establish internal procedures and responsible parties for collecting required documents regularly.

DATA COLLECTION

Data collection and its organization begin early in the accreditation process. Faculty, administrators, and others involved in accreditation should gather pertinent documents, both internal and external, related to each of the standards and respective key elements. One office should serve as the administrator of this data and information, even if some is duplicated in other offices. This approach is useful, even after major accreditation reviews, for correspondence with external agencies, such as state boards of nursing, and as there are changes to faculty and staff.

Our Process

Rather than having standards groups responsible for collecting data related to their standards, the editors were responsible for collecting all the data and documentation (such as syllabi, faculty curricula vitae [CVs], etc.). They would request relevant documents from committees, program directors, and faculty/staff across the school and university, as is needed. Assigning one to two individuals as the data custodians for the project minimized the number of requests to offices outside of the school. As the self-study editors were already the custodians of relevant school data, such as alumni surveys, student satisfaction reports, faculty outcomes, employment data, and certification pass rates, they led this effort. The student services and campus institutional research offices provided further data on student enrollment trends and grievances. With the assistance of these offices, we gathered all of the internal and external reports, which served as the foundation for the self-study report.

WRITING THE SELF-STUDY

The self-study report is an opportunity to involve many faculty and staff from the school of nursing to work as a team. The emphasis is to read each standard and key element carefully and capture enthusiastic points of pride along with data on accomplishments.

Our Process

As mentioned earlier in the chapter, we formed writing groups to increase faculty and staff involvement. Each standard and its key elements were facilitated by program directors. Our goal was to "get it on paper" and then edit as necessary later. We focused on the analysis of data we had collected because this is critical to the success of the self-study, and it gave context and meaning to all evidence. The final submission included an electronic copy of the self-study document (including appendices), a program information form, an agenda, and verification of the opportunity to selected stakeholders for their review and comments.

It is important to note that self-study reports rely heavily on technical writing, and answering each standard clearly and succinctly. We included a glossary at the beginning of our self-study report; this helps evaluators both while reading the self-study and as they conduct the site visit as different schools use their own unique acronyms or abbreviations. Evaluation teams are generally responsible for determining if a program is compliant or noncompliant within each standard and key element. Having significant success in a standard related to employment outcomes, for instance, may not preclude a school from documenting compliance concerning curriculum approval processes. The writing group facilitators and project managers of the self-study process must, therefore, ensure each standard is addressed fully. Box 7.2 provides tips for writing groups and editors to keep in mind as they draft the self-study report.

PREPARING FOR A SITE VISIT

Faculty and administrators should plan for the site team visit at least 6 to 12 months in advance including planning for travel and accommodations and getting to know the site team visitors. The site visit planning should commence as soon as visit dates are confirmed. The school of nursing is responsible for paying for the flights, transportation, and hotel accommodations. The person assigned to transport evaluation team members serves as the initial ambassador for your school and should be prepared to answer detailed questions about its program offerings, internal processes, and more. It is important that all internal and external stakeholders recognize that each interaction is part of the site visit, including any breaks between meetings and transporting the evaluators to and from clinical agencies. Whoever is coordinating the site visit should inquire about specific needs of the team members, such as mobility. Housing should be at a comfortable and convenient location near the school, as the team members must be able to come and go without difficulty. In addition, the school should meticulously organize the document room, whether digital or physical, where evidentiary materials are stored.

Our Process

We started planning for the site team visit 12 months in advance by creating a step-by-step schedule, which included all the on-site members and their specific duties. We reached out to university leadership, community partners, and school leadership with save-the-dates for the site visit. We planned for each team member to be picked up at

BOX 7.2

Tips for Writing Self-Study

1. Carefully review and follow any provided templates and required documentation.
2. Focus on evidence and analysis.
3. Gather evidence of continuous improvement based on accreditation standards and values of the accrediting body and school of nursing (address any methods used to gather evidence in informing improvement efforts; include well-selected evidence).
4. Gather data in a meaningful way for the nursing program (data that are continuous, not episodic).
5. Document the process and the data collected for future accreditation reviews.
6. Organize the report by standard and key elements. As each draft is compiled, identify the following for each standard and key element:
   a. Strengths
   b. Areas of improvement
   c. Action plans
7. Be selective in including any tables or graphs, they should be relevant to the standard and narrative. Such as:
   a. Program completion rates
   b. Graduate outcomes: licensure rates, employment rates
   c. Faculty listing
   d. Faculty outcome data: publications, presentations, etc.
8. If applicable: Address distance education programs
   a. Equipment and technology
   b. Faculty preparation to teach online courses
   c. Student access to support services and resources
   d. Student outcomes versus the traditional on-campus program
   e. Other pertinent information
9. Include evidence in self-study or appendices referring to the resource room materials, when appropriate.
10. In organizing appendices, consider your audience: relate to self-study documents and resource room materials, and include tables and graphs.
11. Be mindful of the length of the report, format, and flow.

the airport at various times. We ensured that accommodations were comfortable, and the location was close to the university for convenient visitor transportation. Since we were aware that the team would continue its work into the evening, we chose a hotel venue that included internet access, a printer, and a meeting space large enough to accommodate a small group. In addition, we recommended that our faculty and staff learn the site team members' credentials ahead of time, for example, current role, clinical expertise, and research and publications.

We held group viewing sessions of accreditation workshops and zoom conference sessions with faculty, staff, and student groups to review the school's mission, vision, and key points of pride. Key points of pride, including employment and licensure rates, were shared with university leaders and community partners. We hosted meetings with committees and other groups at one month and one week before the visit to discuss what to expect during the meeting sessions and answer any pending questions.

Transitioning to Virtual Site Visits

Six months before our most recently scheduled on-site visit, the accrediting agency notified us that our visit would be changed to a virtual visit due to the COVID-19 pandemic. The visit would remain largely the same, with the same number of days allotted and the same number of team members. It was expected that evaluators would still be able to meet virtually with community partners, observe classroom instruction, and tour facilities. With the advent of virtual conferencing applications, it is possible virtual site visits may continue long past the unexpected needs of operating in a pandemic. Virtual site visits allow evaluators to join a review from different time zones and cost significantly less for schools and colleges, as there are no expenses associated with transportation, food, or lodging.

As much as possible, schools should treat the visit as if evaluators were on-site for the review. Key faculty, staff, and administrators should block their calendars so that they are available for the duration of the visit, much like they would for an on-site visit. Assign virtual hosts for meetings and be deliberate in who you choose. Much like an on-site visit, evaluators will speak to their hosts before and after meetings, asking questions, making requests, etc. Virtual hosts can begin the calls, introduce campus representatives, take attendance, and troubleshoot. Work with your IT department in choosing a secure cloud-based storage system and video-conferencing application. Programs may need to create new university emails/profiles for the evaluators so that they can access university systems, such as learning management systems, student information systems, and clinical placement software. Be prepared to create a unique login even if you are not planning to use one for each team member. We had an evaluator who was unable to access any systems with their personal email address after the first day. We created a university login for them with access limited to the duration of the visit. Agendas for virtual visits should be carefully crafted so that only those attending a meeting have access to the video conference links. Your school can reserve conference rooms on-site if desired (and safe) so that evaluators in different locations can virtually meet with or present to on-site groups.

With regard to visiting facilities, we worked with the communications and marketing team to create video tours of our facilities and reached out to our partner facilities to provide the same. Cameras were already set up in our classrooms for video conferencing and remote access during the pandemic and we used these for evaluators to virtually attend class sessions during their review (Vergara & Clochesy, 2021).

DOCUMENT ROOM ORGANIZATION

While historically, resource rooms were used to house all materials and documentation evaluators would review during their visit, we used a digital resource room due to the virtual site visit. This is the way most schools/colleges store such documents already, using cloud-based software. Essentially, we created a filing system on a cloud-based server that was reserved solely for the site visit team as the virtual resource room and organized as such, as opposed to giving evaluators access to all school folders. The digital resource room should be reserved for the evaluators and select faculty and staff to minimize the risk of documents being edited or moved. By creating a unique digital resource room, we could provide copies of internal school documents without providing access to all school files.

Even if returning to live visits or hybrid visits, a digital resource room can and should be used if allowed by the site visit team. Many reviewers prefer documents to be available electronically either way. For the document room, you should have a physical and/or digital environment that allows the site team to easily locate and review necessary documents. It is important to create an index or resource room guide that directs the site visitors to where they can locate all materials. The digital index can include hyperlinks to each document within the resource room. This assists greatly with any documentation that is needed across several standards. For instance, program handbooks were referenced in two standards. A school can organize their resource room index/guide by standard, and documentation by category. For instance, program handbooks can be listed with hyperlinks under the appropriate standards in the index, as well as available by browsing the resource room for the folder, Program Handbooks. Each evaluator will have their individual preference for reviewing materials and using this strategy will help tremendously during the visit.

If the visit is on-site, a physical workspace should be well-lit, quiet, and private. Sufficient office supplies should be placed in the room for each of the evaluators, including a printer and other requirements of the accrediting body. The workspace should be a location that allows easy access to other resources in the school of nursing, including the main administrative offices and restrooms. The space does not have to be elaborate but should contain a large surface for reviewing materials. The document room is a visual display of materials that allows the team to understand how your nursing program meets their accreditation standards. The room also serves as a centralized location for the team to leave their belongings, review materials, and conduct executive sessions. Information technology staff should be readily available throughout the visit for any technical difficulties that may arise. We provided evaluators with a cheat sheet of contacts for any information technology (IT) assistance they might need (i.e., questions, and general troubleshooting). Any on-site evaluators should be provided with a go-to contact for transportation and food or refreshment needs.

Our Process

We were particular with our document room organization. We selected a room that was quiet and well-lit, provided a large surface area for spreading out material, and allowed for writing and keyboarding access. The physical space should be large enough for the team to accommodate their laptops and any documents for review, and with enough space so that team members can meet as a team. While we were cognizant that most evaluators travel with their own laptops, we reserved laptops with Internet access and printers for the site team visitors. We created a resource room guide for the visitors to easily locate the materials we had referenced in our self-study document. On-site resource room documents can be bound in file binders and color-coded, as well as available electronically. We believe that this plan, although redundant, allows for different preferences among the site team and eases their workflow.

We included the following documents in the resource room:

> Faculty CV consistently formatted to allow for ease of reading.

> University reports: Copies of all pertinent reports were made available, including university accreditation documents, such as the Southern Association for Colleges and Schools Commission on Colleges (SACSCOC), and all related assessment and program reports.

> Minutes from all college of nursing committees.

> Correspondence: copies of all correspondence with the accrediting body and other major institutional accreditors.

> Examples of student work.

> Program handbooks.

> Faculty manuals.

> School of nursing bylaws.

> Evaluation data and currently used forms, including student, alumni, employer, and other constituent survey instruments, and summaries/analyses of survey responses.

Many of these documents may be required by the accrediting body. Schools should be sure to review any guidelines or resource manuals carefully as they ready the document room (virtual or otherwise). On-site documents can be filed in three-ring binders and color-coordinated for each level and option of the undergraduate and graduate nursing programs. For example, the undergraduate program should be organized with all syllabi located logically from front to back. Examples of class assignments and student work are placed within each binder to highlight successful attainment of university, program, and/or course outcomes. The self-study report selectively highlighted specific examples of individual courses and carefully cross-referenced meeting minutes, course syllabi, and student examples. We believe it is important to cross-reference examples from the self-study document and have materials easily followed with links to electronic and/or paper evidence. For example, if we discussed a curricular change, we documented where the initial idea originated (e.g., from national standards or research data, or feedback from students or communities of interest) and then tracked the progress of that idea through our processes to final implementation and evaluation. Box 7.3 provides tips for planning the document room.

POTENTIAL PROBLEMS AND CHALLENGES

Problems may arise if the school is not prepared to address the questions from the team. You should have one person assigned to be the nursing program lead. This person is the primary contact for organizing the visit and may be the dean, director, chair, or another individual. You should plan in advance and have examples of materials the team might ask for, for example, previous reports of licensure pass rates, course evaluations, or copies of agency contracts. It is important to be clear in the report about gap areas you might need to improve on and how the school is addressing them.

BOX 7.3

Tips for Planning Document Room

Communicate preliminary planning details with only the team leader.

Assign one person in charge of all communication with the visiting team via the team leader, as well as for arranging transportation and accommodations for the accreditation team.

Arrange for transportation of team members from the first day they arrive until they leave.

Each communication is vital and may contribute to the report; select the correct person for each task.

Begin preparing the document room 6 months in advance.

Be organized and consider using three-ring binders that have clear labels and numbers on the outside of the binder edge for ease of location.

Have a clear index with all pages numbered consistently.

Cross-reference documents by binder number and page.

Label documents consistently.

Make the process of finding examples easy for the team (for example, if you are discussing a change in course objectives, follow your own internal process, demonstrate the votes that occurred in each committee, and provide copies of the minutes and decisions. That way the site reviewer can identify how you followed the proper process to discuss and approve curricular changes).

Provide both written and electronic documents.

Be certain all links for online documents are current and active.

Provide office supplies, including a printer and paper for team use in the resource room.

Assign one person responsible for all formatting and final submission.

Another possible area of concern is when your community of interest, including students, is not adequately prepared for the site visit. Students, agencies, and colleagues in the parent institution need to understand the purpose of the site team visit and how the school of nursing will be responding. You can send emails and letters to the community of interest explaining the accreditation process, their role, and the dates of the site visit. It is important to point out the vital role of all members of the community in validating data and outcomes of the school of nursing. There should be one contact person in the school of nursing designated to reply to questions.

Students and staff should be engaged at least six months in advance and taught about the terminology the team might use so they can answer any questions honestly and clearly. Staff members should be engaged early on as they may be called upon during the visit to meet with team members and provide further information about program operations. Nursing student leaders can become active members in preparing for the site visit and can teach other students about terms the accreditation team might use and why the accreditation process is important.

Summary

This chapter described the process of preparing for the accreditation site visit at our school. It is important that faculty and staff in schools of nursing work as a team at least 18 to 24 months prior to the visit to prepare for the site visit. Other strategies we used were provided in this chapter.

References

National League for Nursing Commission for Nursing Education Accreditation. (2021). *Accreditation standards for nursing education programs*. https://cnea.nln.org/standards-of-accreditation

Vergara, D., & Clochesy, J. M. (2021). Preparing for and hosting virtual regulatory and accreditation site visits. *Nurse Educator, 46*(6), 334–335. doi: 10.1097/NNE.0000000000001027

8

Assessment of Online Courses and Programs

Karen H. Frith, PhD, RN, NEA-BC, CNE

Assessment of online courses and programs is an integral part of a nursing program's systematic program evaluation plan for continuous improvement and accreditation. Since the early 2000s, online education has been a viable method for educating students in nursing programs. However, the COVID-19 pandemic caused it to become the *only* method for educating students for many months. This sudden shift in modality thrust faculty into learning about technologies and using them creatively to replace the classroom, laboratory, and clinical experiences, when necessary. Faculty wrote about their experiences, and more research literature about online education is now available. This chapter addresses evaluating online courses, establishing benchmarks for program success, and assessing the quality of courses and programs using valid and reliable tools. Finally, the chapter describes the issues surrounding online nursing courses and programs offered in other states and the impact on evaluation and accreditation.

EVALUATION IN AN ONLINE ENVIRONMENT

Accreditation

Administrators of online programs must provide resources to support educationally sound courses that produce outcomes like courses offered on campus (Frith, 2020a, 2020b). This premise reflects the standards for evaluation of online programs in nursing from regional accrediting organizations, such as the Middle States Commission on Higher Education and Southern Association of Colleges and Schools Commission on Colleges, and nursing accreditation bodies, including the Accreditation Commission for Education in Nursing (ACEN), Commission on Collegiate Nursing Education (CCNE), and Commission for Nursing Education Accreditation (CNEA).

The National Council for State Authorization Reciprocity Agreements (NC-SARA) released its guidelines on distance education, *21st Century Distance Education Guidelines,* for evaluating online education programs in nursing (NC-SARA, 2021). The guidelines include institutional capacity, institutional transparency, disclosures, academic programs, student support, program review, and academic and institutional integrity. The 2021 guidelines, compared to the 2011 guidelines, have a stronger emphasis on transparency, institutional disclosures to students, and academic integrity.

Institutional capacity means the postsecondary and higher education institutions must maintain "financial resources, technology infrastructure, data security, content expertise, instructional design, support for students and assessment of, and access to information resources" (NC-SARA, 2021, p. 4). The institution must provide appropriate financial, human, and technology resources to sustain high-quality courses and programs. In other words, distance education must be part of the institution's mission and strategic goals.

The consumer protection guidelines require disclosure about the curriculum, student learning outcomes, and program outcomes, including rates for passing licensure and certification examinations, graduation, and employment. The guidelines also require institutions to protect students by disclosing the costs of tuition, institution fees, books, software, materials, identification or proctoring services, travel, and clinical experiences. The institution also should communicate its refund policies to prospective and enrolled students. It must disclose the need for prerequisite courses, technology, internet connection speed, and expected student engagement per week.

The institution should have faculty with subject-matter expertise responsible for delivering the online learning curricula and evaluating the students' success in achieving the learning outcomes, should engage in regular program evaluation, and should use the results of its evaluations to improve the quality of academic offerings and student services. The institution should provide student orientation to technology and academic support services, equivalent to on-campus student services. Finally, the institution should encourage a culture of academic integrity and invest in methods to detect instances of academic misconduct. The entire document is available for review at https://www.c-rac.org/post/c-rac-statement-on-nc-sara-distance-education-guidelines. In addition to the guidelines, the NC-SARA maintains a searchable index of state requirements, including authorization of distance education, physical presence policy, student complaints, tuition refund policy, student tuition recovery fund, reporting, enforcement, and the application process. Readers can find the index at https://www.nc-sara.org/guide/state-authorization-guide.

Colleges, universities, or other education institutions might seek the Distance Education Accrediting Commission (DEAC) accreditation. The accreditation process requires the completion of training materials, applications, and fees. To be eligible for accreditation, the institution must have been operating as a legal entity for two years and enrolling students for one year. An institution applying for initial accreditation first must be assessed for readiness by an independent DEAC-appointed evaluator; if the DEAC evaluator finds the institution eligible, then it submits a self-evaluation report. The DEAC Accreditation Manual (DEAC, 2021) and Online Training Center (DEAC, 2022) guide institutions that are seeking accreditation.

The accreditation organizations in nursing have accreditation standards that address distance education. CCNE integrates requirements for distance education into all standards and key elements (CCNE, 2018). The *ACEN Accreditation Manual Section II: Policies* (ACEN, 2020) provide a list of the most critical elements of online program quality and a detailed description of the quality elements. The manual states that online programs need to be congruent with the institution's mission. The institution must use appropriate and evidence-based instructional design methods for the mode of delivery, and the faculty should evaluate the achievement of student learning outcomes. The institution needs to have competent online faculty who are subject matter experts with access to technical support services. The institution must have high-quality, accessible student support services and a reliable method for student identification through the student enrollment life cycle. The faculty who teach in the online program should use accessible, current, and relevant learning resources appropriate to the modality. Lastly, it is important for faculty to have regular interactions with students in each course and build these into the course design.

Instructional Design

The NC-SARA Guidelines (2021) and ACEN Manual (2020) require the design and delivery of online courses to enable communication and active participation of students with each other and their faculty members. The design of online courses and the choice of teaching approaches should be a concern for any nursing program. The Quality Matters (QM) Higher Education Rubric is a widely used tool for evaluating the overall course design (QM, 2020). Evaluation using the QM Rubric focuses on the alignment of elements of the course with each other to achieve desired student outcomes. Faculty can engage in peer evaluation using the rubric or request review by the QM peer review team.

Interface Design

The interface design concerns the usability of the learning management system or other online technologies to minimize the cognitive load on students, making the system effective, efficient, and satisfying for students (International Organization for Standardization, 2021). Even though faculty do not design their learning management systems, they often serve on a product selection committee. Knowledge of usability can assist faculty in evaluating and selecting a learning management system that is user-friendly for students and faculty.

Navigation Design

Faculty and instructional designers control navigation design within a learning management system. Most learning management systems are flexible enough to allow faculty to organize their courses in different ways; however, this flexibility can create a barrier to learning if navigation is different from course to course in an online program. Faculty involved in an online program should evaluate the navigation design across all courses in the program. If navigation is different, faculty can develop navigation templates for their online courses to standardize them in collaboration with instructional designers.

Content Design

Innovations in technology and the adoption of technologies into online course offerings can be overwhelming to faculty who must keep current in nursing practice and scholarship. Faculty are content experts in the courses they teach, but they may need a consultation with instructional designers to improve the online delivery of content to students. However, instructional designers who are up to date on adopting new technologies for pedagogical reasons make excellent partners for faculty content experts. For example, a faculty member teaching a course on evidence-based practice (EBP) could simply use an EBP model to organize the content and provide textbooks and articles for students to read to learn the material. However, the faculty member could also deliver content using synchronous video conferencing, asynchronous discussion boards, games, and other methods to increase interactivity and communication. Further, the faculty member could use collaborative groups for learning activities and assignments so they learn together and increase a sense of connection to each other.

Evaluation

Formative

Faculty should design evaluations for every online course. As students move through the content, data about student performance at the course level can automatically be generated through quizzes, discussion forums, polls, and other methods. Faculty should use formative assessments to provide feedback to students as they are learning, not as a graded activity (Frith, 2020a, 2020b). As with any formative evaluation, faculty can use the data to clarify misunderstood concepts or guide students to a deeper understanding. In addition, faculty can use formative evaluation to take corrective action in the design of the course during its delivery or before the next offering.

Summative

Research has shown consistently that students who take online courses perform as well and sometimes slightly better than students in campus-based courses and are satisfied with online courses (Castro & Tumibay, 2021; He et al., 2021). Student achievement of learning outcomes and satisfaction is necessary to evaluate every course. Other summative evaluations appropriate to online courses can include the time students spend on modules or assignments, the need for technical support for activities or assignments, academic misconduct or student identity problems, and the effectiveness of course learning activities on final grades.

Formative and summative evaluations are of little value unless faculty use the data to adjust instruction or improve future course offerings. Therefore, formative and summative data from online courses, the actions taken by faculty, and resulting outcomes serve as complete cycles of improvement. Documentation of improvements can be saved in course books for accreditation and presented to a curriculum committee to stimulate improvements across an online program.

ASSESSING QUALITY OF COURSES AND PROGRAMS

A closely related concept to summative evaluation is assessing the quality of online courses and programs. Whereas summative evaluation focuses on students' performance in a course and their satisfaction with that course, assessing the quality of online courses and programs is a formal process for measuring indicators, using the data to develop an improvement plan, and reassessing indicators to determine effectiveness. A nursing program might fold the online assessment plan into comprehensive evaluation plans for on-campus programs or set them apart. In either case, faculty and program administrators work together to design an assessment plan that leads to continuous improvement and data-driven decision-making.

There are several widely used frameworks for assessing quality in online education, including the Online Learning Consortium Quality Framework (OLC, 2022) and Quality Matters (QM, 2020). (Anstey and Watson, 2018) created a comprehensive rubric for evaluating educational technology used in online education. The rubric has eight major categories with several criteria per category. The categories include functionality; accessibility; technical; mobile design; privacy, data protection, and rights; social presence; teaching presence; and cognitive presence. Readers can find the free rubric at https://teaching.uwo.ca/pdf/elearning/Rubric-for-eLearning-Tool-Evaluation.pdf. Castro and Tumibay (2021) derived a conceptual framework from a literature review about online learning. This framework identifies factors that contribute to quality online courses, including teaching strategies, course design, institutional support, and the characteristics of faculty and students (Fig. 8.1).

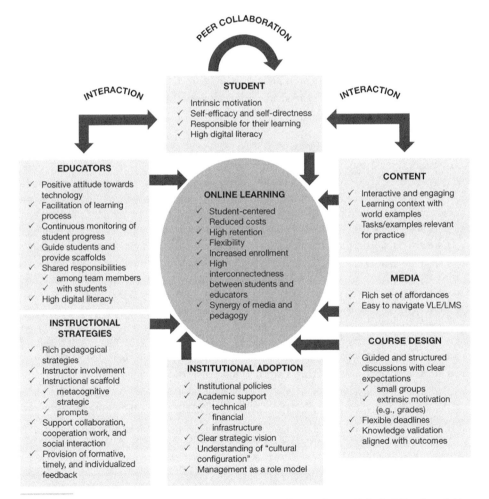

FIGURE 8.1 A conceptual diagram of online learning factors. Source: Castro, M. D. B., & Tumibay, G. M. (2021). A literature review: Efficacy of online learning courses for higher education institution using meta-analysis. *Education and Information Technologies, 26*(2), 1382. https://doi.org/10.1007/s10639-019-10027-z. Reprinted by permission, Springer Nature, 2022.

A nursing program can adapt a framework for assessing quality in online courses and programs by selecting representative indicators from each part of a framework. Once the framework and indicators are selected, the quality improvement plan can include indicators, benchmarks, data sources, persons responsible for assessment, frequency of assessment, actual outcomes, action plan, and action result. The plan guides faculty and administrators to be deliberate in their approach to quality improvement.

Benchmarks for Program Success

Benchmarks are the expected outcomes set by faculty and administrators which indicate the program is successful. Nursing programs might set benchmarks, such as retention and graduation rates, licensure and certification pass rates, student engagement scores, student satisfaction with the course and support services, and technical support report to resolution time. If the actual outcome falls short of the benchmark, then the faculty and administrators would act and reassess the indicator. Table 8.1 provides an improvement plan with a benchmark of 90% persistence in online courses and a benchmark of 80% graduation in an online program. The following section on tools provides the measurement of subjective indicators used as benchmarks.

Tools

Nursing programs often use college- or university-developed tools to measure progress toward benchmarks for an entirely online program. As an internal measurement, these tools work well if used to trend performance over time. However, faculty offering online courses who wish to compare their programs to similar programs or conduct research can use published tools with normed scores and established validity and reliability statistics.

There are published tools that measure a philosophical approach to online education. The Community of Inquiry (CoI) Framework (Garrison et al., 2020) focuses on three types of presence in online education: teaching, social, and cognitive presence. Arbaugh and colleagues (2008) developed the CoI Instrument, a valid and reliable tool, to measure the three types of presence. The tool contains 34 items, and factor analysis using principal components analysis and oblique rotation yielded three subscales. The subscales are reliable as shown by internal consistency (Cronbach's alpha) of 0.94 in the teaching presence subscale, 0.91 in the social presence subscale, and 0.95 in the cognitive presence subscale (Arbaugh et al., 2008). Faculty have used the CoI framework and tools for over two decades. If interested in learning more about the research evidence supporting the design and evaluation of online courses using the CoI, nurse educators should review the article by Fiock (2020).

Nursing programs that use a constructivist pedagogy stress learning as interaction with existing knowledge and new knowledge through engagement. Programs with such a focus might use the National Survey of Student Engagement (NSSE). The NSSE does not focus on online education per se. However, the NSSE reports ten engagement indicators important to online education, including academic challenges, learning with peers, experiences with faculty, and campus environment (Center for Postsecondary Research, 2021). The items are scored on a 0–60 scale with answer options of never (0 points), sometimes (20 points), often (40 points), and very often (60 points). A mean

TABLE 8.1

Example of Plan for Measuring Quality in Distance Education Courses and Programs

Assessment Indicator	Benchmark for Success	Data Sources	Responsible	Schedule	Location of Document	Actual Outcomes	Action Plan	Action Result
Persistence in MSN online courses	90% of students registered for an online course complete the course	Information system for student records	Advisor, program director, curriculum committee	At the end of each semester	Table of quality measurements reported in the curriculum committee minutes	85% of students in fall semester completed online courses. 10% of students never logged into the learning management system (LMS) across all courses.	The curriculum committee voted to require orientation at the beginning of each semester for all online courses. Faculty agreed to send a list of students who had not logged into the LMS after the first 3 days of the semester to the advisor for follow-up.	In spring semester, 92% of students completed courses with only 3% never having logged into the LMS Recommend: Continue monitoring and advisor follow-up.
Graduation rates in the MSN online program	80% of students enrolled in the online MSN program complete the program in 8 semesters.	Information system for student records and MSN database	Advisor, program director, curriculum committee	Yearly after graduation	Table of quality measurements reported in the curriculum committee minutes	78% of students who enrolled in the first MSN online course completed the online program	The advisor and program director will use an early warning system to track continued registration of students who start the online MSN program. Students who have not registered within 2 weeks of the start of registration will be contacted by email or telephone.	The follow-up with students at registration revealed that most students who had not registered were waiting until financial aid was available. The program director will work with the offices of financial aid and registrar to look for solutions. Recommend: Continue monitoring with early warning system.

is calculated in each of the four engagement categories and then weighted based on demographics in the sample. The validity and reliability of the NSSE are extensively documented. Other research instruments measure student engagement, such as the *Online Student Engagement* (Dixson, 2015) and the *Student Experience in the Research University* (Bae & Han, 2019).

Nursing programs that use the Seven Principles of Good Practices in Undergraduate Programs (Chickering & Gamson, 1987) as the framework for their online programs could use a survey created by Crews, Wilkinson, and Neill (2015). The survey contains 36 items with Likert-type answer options. All items are matched to the seven principles. The survey authors did not offer any reliability assessments, but the tool has face validity. Faculty could easily adapt the survey for nursing programs.

ONLINE PROGRAMS OFFERED ACROSS STATES
State Authorization

State governments have the authority to authorize higher education degrees or courses offered within their boundaries. The approval process includes degrees and courses offered on-campus and degrees and courses offered through online technologies. The United States Department of Education issued Title 34, §600.9(c) requiring an institution offering postsecondary education through distance or correspondence education to meet state requirements (Code of Federal Regulation, 2022).

The cost of state authorization on institutions of higher education that offer online courses and degrees is high. Institutions can hire personnel to monitor state laws and regulations and seek state governments approval. Fees charged by state governments vary, making institutional planning difficult. These problems have been complex for both higher education institutions and state governments. In response to the problems associated with state authorization, the four regional education compacts (Midwestern Higher Education Compact, New England Board of Higher Education, Southern Regional Education Board, and Western Interstate Commission for Higher Education) established a cooperative agreement, the State Authorization Reciprocity Agreement (NC-SARA, 2021). One of the purposes of SARA is to make state authorization more efficient and less burdensome on higher education institutions and states. Other purposes of SARA include giving guidance on accreditation and institutional quality to avoid redundancy in accreditation requirements, providing a means for consumer protection, and defining institutional financial responsibility to avoid additional regulations for online education (SARA).

States interested in enrollment in SARA must first be members of a regional education compact. Once a member, the state can enroll in SARA. The enrollment process began in January 2014; as of this writing, there are 49 states in SARA (National Council for State Authorization Reciprocity Agreements) (NC-SARA, 2021). Readers should access the SARA Manual for more information (https://nc-sara.org/sites/default/files/files/2021-05/SARA_Policy_Manual_21.1.pdf).

Even though SARA provides a more consistent and streamlined approach to state authorization for institutions in member states, higher education institutions with nursing programs have additional requirements because of state boards of nursing (NC-SARA, 2021). Institutions that offer online courses or degree programs leading to professional licensure are required to keep prospective students informed about state licensing requirements by providing such information in writing. If the institution cannot confirm whether the course or degree meets the requirements for professional licensure in a prospective student's state, the institution is required to provide the student with current contact information for the state board of nursing in which the student lives (NC-SARA).

National Council of State Boards of Nursing

The National Council of State Boards of Nursing (NCSBN) issued a white paper on nursing regulation of distance education, which provided background information about online education, definitions, and general guidance for state boards of nursing (NCSBN, 2015). Two key definitions for the general guidelines are home and host state/jurisdictions. The home state/jurisdiction is "where the distance education program has a legal domicile, and the host state/jurisdiction is the state/jurisdiction outside of the home state/jurisdiction where students participate in didactic coursework and clinical experiences" (NCSBN, 2015, p. 2). The NCSBN proposed the following guidelines for distance education prelicensure nursing education programs:

> Programs shall meet the same approval guidelines as any other prelicensure program in the home state;
> The home state/jurisdiction approves prelicensure nursing education programs, including distance learning education programs;
> Programs in the home state provide oversight over the students in the host states and are responsible for the students' supervision;
> Faculty, preceptors, or others who teach clinical experiences should hold a current and active nursing license or privilege to practice, which is not encumbered, and meet licensure requirements in the state where the patient is located. Faculty who teach didactic content for a prelicensure nursing education program using distance education shall hold a current and active nursing license or privilege to practice, which is not encumbered, and meet licensure requirements in the home state where the program is approved; and
> State Boards of Nursing will communicate information through their annual reports about prelicensure nursing programs with students enrolled in clinical experiences in host states (NCSBN, 2015, p. 7–9).

The NCSBN hosts a web page on prelicensure distance education requirements for the states and territories at https://www.ncsbn.org/13663.htm and a page on Advanced Practice distance education requirements at https://www.ncsbn.org/13662.htm (NCSBN, 2022a, 2022b). Some state boards of nursing require extensive approvals, while others have few requirements. For example, a nursing program with distance education offerings whose "home state" is Georgia could have a student living in and wanting clinical experiences in Arizona (host state). In this case, the nursing program would check the NCSBN website and find that Arizona's regulations require the following:

> A self-study, describing the program's compliance with the Board's standards for organization, administration, resources, facilities, services, records, faculty and administrator qualifications, policies, and curriculum.

➤ A statement of the number and type of planned clinical placements, and copies of contracts and commitments with the planned clinical facilities.

➤ Names and qualifications of Arizona-licensed and physically present supervising faculty.

➤ Verification of the program's good standing in the home state (NCSBN, 2022a).

If the student lived in and wanted clinical experiences in Virginia as the "host state," there are no regulations by the Virginia State Board of Nursing. The lack of standard requirements for all state boards of nursing adds to the confusion and costs for nursing programs offering distance education.

Contracts for Clinical Affiliations

Nursing education programs offering online courses with clinical experiences must check the regulations for each state in which students plan to do their clinical experiences before sending clinical affiliation contracts to health care agencies in the host state. Even when a nursing program gets state board of nursing approval, getting the host state's health care agencies to sign clinical affiliation contracts usually takes months and may not be successful. Because of the long period to obtain a clinical affiliation contract, nursing programs should begin the process upon admission or early in the student's enrollment in an online course or program.

Assessment of online courses and programs follows similar strategies used for campus-based education, including concern for accreditation and quality improvement. The assessment can be designed as a stand-alone process or integrated into a nursing program's comprehensive assessment plan. Faculty and administrators with programmatic responsibility for online courses and programs have the added responsibility for compliance with regulatory requirements from host states and the boards of nursing. A systematic program evaluation plan based on a continuous improvement model in online education can be a nursing program's best asset to maintain quality in all offerings.

Summary

Institutions with online programs need to provide resources to support educationally sound courses that result in outcomes similar to courses offered on campus. This premise reflects the standards for evaluation of online programs from regional accrediting organizations, such as the Middle States Commission on Higher Education, and accreditation organizations in nursing.

There are several widely used frameworks for assessing quality in online education, including the OLC and QM, discussed in this chapter. As part of program evaluation, nursing programs set benchmarks, such as retention and graduation rates. These benchmarks are the expected outcomes that indicate the program is successful regardless of whether the program is offered online or on campus.

Assessment of online courses and programs follows similar strategies used for campus-based education, including concern for accreditation and quality improvement. The assessment can be designed as a stand-alone process or integrated into a nursing program's comprehensive assessment plan. Faculty and administrators with programmatic responsibility for online courses and programs have the added responsibility for compliance with regulatory requirements from host states and boards of nursing. A systematic program evaluation plan based on a continuous improvement model in online education can be a nursing program's best asset to maintain quality in all offerings.

References

Accreditation Commission for Education in Nursing (ACEN). (2020). *ACEN accreditation manual-Section II*. Retrieved June 13, 2022, from https://www.acenursing.org/accreditation-manual-policies/

Anstey, L., & Watson, G. (2018). *Rubric for eLearning Tool Evaluation*. Western University. https://teaching.uwo.ca/pdf/elearning/Rubric-for-eLearning-Tool-Evaluation.pdf

Arbaugh, J. B., Cleveland-Innes, M., Diaz, S. R., Garrison, D. R., Ice, P., Richardson, J. C., & Swan, K. P. (2008). Developing a community of inquiry instrument: Testing a measure of the Community of Inquiry framework using a multi-institutional sample. Part of a special section of the AERA Education and World Wide Web Special Interest Group (EdWeb/SIG), *11*(3/4), 133–136. doi:10.1016/j.iheduc.2008.06.003

Bae, Y., & Han, S. (2019). Academic engagement and learning outcomes of the student experience in the research university: Construct validation of the instrument. *Educational Sciences: Theory & Practice, 19*(3), 49–64.

Castro, M. D. B., & Tumibay, G. M. (2021). A literature review: Efficacy of online learning courses for higher education institution using meta-analysis. *Education and Information Technologies, 26*(2), 1367–1385. https://doi.org/10.1007/s10639-019-10027-z

Center for Postsecondary Research. (2021). *National Survey of Student Engagement (NSSE)*. Evidence-based improvement in higher education. https://nsse.indiana.edu//nsse/about-nsse/index.html

Chickering, A. W., & Gamson, Z. F. (1987). Seven principles for good practices in undergraduate education. *American Association of Higher Education Bulletin, 39*(7), 3–6.

Code of Federal Regulations. (2022). 34 CFR § 600.9 State authorization.

Commission on Collegiate Nursing Education (CCNE). (2018). *CCNE: Standards, procedures & guidelines*. https://www.aacnnursing.org/CCNE-Accreditation/Accreditation-Resources/Standards-Procedures-Guidelines

Crews, T., Wilkinson, K., & Neill, J. (2015). Principles for good practice in undergraduate education: Effective online course design to assist students' success. *MERLOT Journal of Online Learning and Teaching, 11*(1), 87–103.

Distance Education Accrediting Commission (DEAC). (2021). *DEAC accreditation handbook*. https://www.deac.org/Seeking-Accreditation/The-DEAC-Accrediting-Handbook.aspx

Distance Education Accreditation Commission (DEAC). (2022). *DEAC. Online training center*. https://www.deactraining.org/

Dixson, M. D. (2015). Measuring student engagement in the online course: The online student engagement scale (OSE). *Online Learning, 19*(4). https://doi.org/10.24059/olj.v19i4.561

Fiock, H. (2020). Designing a community of inquiry in online courses. *The International Review of Research in Open and Distributed Learning, 21*(1), 135–153. https://doi.org/10.19173/irrodl.v20i5.3985

Frith, K. H. (2020a). Assessment of online education: Part 1. *Nursing Education Perspectives, 41*(5), 320–321. https://doi.org/10.1097/01.NEP.0000000000000727

Frith, K. H. (2020b). Assessment of online education: Part 2. *Nursing Education Perspectives, 41*(6), 386–387. https://doi.org/10.1097/01.nep.0000000000000745

Garrison, R., Cleveland-Innes, M., & Vaughan, N. (2020). *Community of Inquiry*. https://coi.athabascau.ca/

He, L., Yang, N., Xu, L., Ping, F., Li, W., Sun, Q., Li, Y., Zhu, H., & Zhang, H. (2021). Synchronous distance education vs traditional education for health science students: A systematic review and meta-analysis. *Medical Education, 55*(3), 293–308. https://doi.org/10.1111/medu.14364

International Organization for Standardization. (2021). ISO Digital Learning Solutions Toolkit. http://www.ios.org.

National Council for State Authorization Reciprocity Agreements (NC-SARA). (2021). *SARA policy manual*. https://nc-sara.org/sites/default/files/files/2021-05/SARA_Policy_Manual_21.1.pdf

National Council for State Authorization Reciprocity, N.-S. (2021). *Proposed 21st century distance education guidelines*. https://www.c-rac.org/post/c-rac-statement-on-distance-education-guidelines

National Council on State Boards of Nursing. (2015). *Nursing regulation recommendations for distance education in prelicensure nursing programs*. https://www.ncsbn.org/cps/rde/xchg/ncsbn/hs.xsl/6662.htm

National Council on State Boards of Nursing. (2022a). *Prelicensure distance education requirements*. https://www.ncsbn.org/13663.htm

National Council on State Boards of Nursing. (2022b). *APRN distance education requirements*. https://www.ncsbn.org/13662.htm

Online Learning Consortium (OLC). (2022). *OLC quality scorecard—improve the quality of online learning & teaching*. OLC. https://onlinelearningconsortium.org/consult/olc-quality-scorecard-suite/

Quality Matters. (2020). *Quality matters higher education rubric* (6th ed.). https://www.qualitymatters.org/qa-resources/rubric-standards

9

Evaluation of Specific Types of Nursing Programs

Joan Such Lockhart, PhD, RN, CNE, FAAN, ANEF

Melinda G. Oberleitner, DNS, RN, FAAN

The COVID-19 pandemic exacerbated an existing nursing shortage (Jacobs, 2021). However, despite concerns that the pandemic would serve as a deterrent to nursing school enrollment, data released by the American Association of Colleges of Nursing (AACN) in early 2021 revealed increases in enrollment in baccalaureate, master's, and doctoral programs in 2020 (AACN, 2021a).

As nursing program administrators scramble to meet societal needs for an ever-increasing supply of nurses at the entry and advanced practice levels, they are often faced with the reality of administering multiple, disparate programs. For example, despite nursing programs often being labeled as expensive to offer, many schools of nursing offer an array of educational tracks and concentrations including programs targeted to prelicensure students with and without previous degrees, RN to Bachelor of Science in Nursing (RN to BSN) programs, RN to Master of Science in Nursing (MSN) programs, master's programs with multiple concentrations, post-master's degree offerings and certificate programs, and programs leading to terminal degrees such as BSN to Doctor of Nursing Practice (DNP), Doctor of Anesthesia Practice (DNAP/DrAP), DNP and Doctor of Philosophy (PhD) programs. As the structure, resource requirements, and outcomes of academic programs are as unique as the graduate that the program is preparing, developing program assessment and evaluation plans with components relevant to each program is critical. This chapter focuses on specific program types and their impact on program assessment and evaluation. Attention is given to select programs to illustrate the need for unique assessment: (1) RN to BSN, (2) accelerated second career, (3) nurse practitioner, (4) nurse anesthetist, and (5) DNP and PhD programs. These areas are important to assess in addition to the typical components of program evaluation discussed in prior chapters.

RN TO BSN PROGRAMS

Although enrollments in RN to BSN programs declined slightly in 2020, approximately 750 RN to BSN programs enrolled over 132,000 students (AACN, 2021b). According to

AACN (2021b), approximately 60% of RN to BSN programs are delivered in online or hybrid formats. Many schools offer accelerated programs in five-, seven-, or eight-week sessions with multiple start dates during the calendar year rather than longer, more traditional semester-based, fall, spring, and summer session offerings. Typical program completion times of students enrolled in RN to BSN programs are between one and two years. To date, there are no national standards or guidelines from national nursing or professional organizations that provide direction for examining program effectiveness related to RN to BSN programs, as accrediting organizations typically evaluate RN to BSN programs within the context of the prelicensure BSN degree program, if one is offered by the school of nursing undergoing accreditation.

Assessment and evaluation of student learning outcomes, although a major and primary component, is but one factor in program evaluation of RN to BSN programs. In the absence of national standards unique to RN to BSN program evaluation, assessment and evaluation of student achievement including retention, progression, and graduation rates, curriculum relevance, and assessment of satisfaction measures should be undertaken with the ultimate goal of using ongoing and systematic evaluation to refine key processes and improve student learning.

Measuring Learning Outcomes

Despite large enrollments in RN to BSN programs nationally, there are limited resources to quantify learning outcomes of RN to BSN students (Wagner et al., 2020). In this article, the authors described a process by which one community college, which offered an RN to BSN program, developed a program outcome measurement tool using Qualtrics software to correlate program objectives with AACN's *The Essentials of Baccalaureate Education for Professional Nursing Practice* (2008). An analysis derived six themes that were used to construct an instrument to measure students' increase in knowledge from program start to end. The final analysis revealed knowledge gains in all thematic areas as assessed from the students' perspective.

Student Progression Tracking

Program assessment and evaluation aspects germane to RN to BSN programs include establishment of benchmarks related to student progression, attrition, retention, and graduation rates. Many schools also track persistence rates of students. However, there is a lack of standardization in definitions of these terms and measurement processes, as well as an absence of national nursing standards related to tracking student progression (Robertson et al., 2010). Accrediting bodies and some state boards of nursing require schools to track graduation rates and may require their own methods of calculation (although many boards of nursing do not regulate post-licensure programs). Thus, it becomes incumbent on nursing faculty and administrators to define important terms and establish reliable term-to-term and year-to-year tracking and comparison methods.

RNs who return to school for their degrees are self-directed individuals who are willing to assume responsibility for achieving an important career goal. However, program flexibility, such as options to complete the program in online and accelerated formats, appear to be key components of degree completion (Matthews & Travis, 1994; O'Brien & Renner, 2000).

Cipher et al. (2017) conducted a retrospective predictive analysis of 9,567 students enrolled in one university's accelerated online RN to BSN program over an eight academic year period to examine demographic and academic predictors of persistence and success as measured by graduation, timely graduation (defined as graduation within six semesters), and discontinuation (defined as no course enrollment for one calendar year). In this analysis, students who were more likely to graduate and to graduate sooner were younger, had previously completed a baccalaureate degree, withdrew from fewer courses, and failed fewer courses. Study authors recommend the creation of an early identification system for high-risk students to inform student recruitment and selection processes.

Curriculum

As stated earlier, there are no national guidelines or recommendations related specifically to the curricular structure of RN to BSN programs or to the unique program-end competencies expected of graduates of these programs. Hooper et al. (2013) presented recommendations for structuring RN to BSN programs. These included ensuring RN to BSN students receive equal course credits as traditional prelicensure students in upper-division nursing and nonnursing courses, requiring a full array of liberal arts courses, and providing course content that was focused directly on role differences of diploma/associate degree nurses and BSN nurses to encompass effective role-transition strategies.

There appears to be consensus in the literature as to which course content should be included in RN to BSN curricula (Baxter, 2018; McEwen et al., 2014; Stokowski, 2011), including content related to leadership/management, community/public health, nursing research/evidence-based practice, and professionalism/legal and ethical issues. Absent any national guidelines related to essential curricular content in RN to BSN programs, these findings may inform content mapping for program assessment and evaluation purposes related to curricular structure.

Linton et al. (2019) described the process one program used to examine gaps between an associate degree in nursing (ADN) program content and AACN's *Essentials for Baccalaureate Education* (AACN, 2008) to reduce redundancy of content and to meet expectations for BSN level education. As part of a three-day off-campus "retreat" and for several months prior to the retreat, faculty examined the results of several measurements including student satisfaction surveys, RN to BSN student learning outcomes evaluation, and outcomes of standardized measurements related to the acquisition of professionalism and cultural competencies. Curriculum mapping was also completed. Gaps in content, such as content addressing health policy, were identified. Subsequently, existing courses were revised or eliminated, and new courses were added to the RN to BSN curriculum. Finally, the faculty compared tuition revenue and student costs of total credit hours in the old and new curriculum plans to determine the financial impact on students.

Recent research has been conducted to determine RN to BSN graduates' perceptions of RN to BSN program curricular content. Sitzman et al. (2020) reported the results of a qualitative narrative survey of 263 RN to BSN students enrolled in the final semester of one university's RN to BSN program between 2016 and 2019 to address the question, "How have you used what you are learning in the RN to BSN program at work?" (p. 267).

Twelve persistent themes emerged from data analysis. The most identified theme by students was gaining new knowledge and confidence to improve clinical practice and patient care by integrating evidence-based practice. Other prominent themes included leadership and professionalism. The authors contend better understanding of content that RN to BSN students find immediately useful in professional practice supports integration of curricular content.

Assuring that the quality of curricula in RN to BSN programs offered in online formats presents additional program evaluation challenges. One well-recognized national organization and program that is committed to ensuring high-quality online course development and delivery is the Quality Matters (QM) program. The QM framework, an example of a faculty-centered peer-review process, can be used by online RN to BSN programs to certify the quality of courses offered in online and hybrid formats and ensure adherence to best practices.

In recognition that greater than 60% of RN to BSN programs are offered in distance learning formats, Perfetto (2019) applied an integrative review methodology to answer the research question, "What are the best practices for distance/online/hybrid RN to BSN program curriculum and instruction?" (p. 18). Emergent themes identified were: (1) relationship of online course design to achievement of learning outcomes and/or student satisfaction, (2) academic integrity in online teaching and learning, (3) experience of community and caring in online courses, and (4) learner characteristics as they relate to success in online courses. Themes identified in this synthesis provide research-based direction to educators offering RN to BSN programs in distance formats as related to program development, evaluation, and improvement.

ACCELERATED BACCALAUREATE IN NURSING PROGRAMS

Accelerated second career programs offer individuals who have completed undergraduate degrees in nonnursing fields with the opportunity to complete their BSN degree in as few as 11 to 18 months (AACN, 2019) or their MSN degree in three years (AACN, 2019). The rapid growth in second career programs helps to alleviate the national nursing shortage by preparing qualified graduates who are ready to enter the nursing workforce in a short time. In addition, accelerated programs help address the Institute of Medicine's (IOM) recommendation to increase the number of BSN nurses to 80% by 2020 (IOM, 2010). While that goal was not realized, the portion of employed RNs who are BSN-prepared or higher has grown by 10% over the decade, from 49% in 2010 to 59% in 2019 (Future of Nursing Campaign for Action, 2021a).

In the United States (US), accelerated bachelor of science in nursing (ABSN) programs have rapidly increased over the past decade. In 2018, 282 programs were in operation and located throughout 49 states, the District of Columbia, Virgin Islands, and Guam, with 30 additional programs in progress (AACN, 2019). Student enrollment figures from ABSN programs also have grown with 23,354 students enrolled in these programs in 2018, an increase of 3,813 students from 2017 (AACN, 2019). Graduation rates have similarly increased from 12,293 to 13,442 during the same one-year time span (AACN, 2019). Growth has also been noted in fast-track options available for students completing their MSN (AACN, 2019) with 64 accelerated or entry-level master's programs in 2018 and 13 programs under development (AACN, 2019).

Accelerated programs must meet the same curriculum standards and accreditation criteria as their traditional BSN and MSN degree counterparts and produce competent graduates prepared to transition to clinical practice. The rapid pace of ABSN programs demands constant attention to assessment and program evaluation efforts with data supporting timely, evidence-based program improvement. While all components of program evaluation are important, ABSN programs in particular require attention to: (1) curriculum and teaching-learning practices, (2) program outcomes, and (3) transition to practice.

Curriculum and Innovative Teaching-Learning Practices

Because ABSN programs target learners who have successfully completed prior degrees, faculty should design curricula that allow students to successfully attain expected learning outcomes in a short period of time. Innovative teaching-learning strategies that are tailored to adult learners and build on their past experiences should be integrated into courses. Schools need to create a supportive environment that fosters effective learning and academic success.

Christoffersen (2017) described several best practices to guide faculty who are new to teaching ABSN students using data obtained via focus groups with 16 experienced faculty and administrators across the US: (1) be prepared and organized; (2) actively engage students in learning and be open to change; (3) foster relationships with students based on mutual respect, active listening, and support; (4) acknowledge work/life experiences; and (5) adopt innovative pedagogy that integrates technology and fosters early immersion into nursing. Consistent with Christoffersen's (2017) recommendations, several authors reported valuable outcomes after implementing innovative approaches with ABSN students, including collaborative testing (Burgess & Medina-Smuck, 2018), flipped classrooms (Shatto et al., 2017), and flipped classrooms and skills labs paired with the Socratic Method (Harlan et al., 2021).

McElwain et al. (2021) adopted an early clinical immersion model (at week four in a 12-month ABSN program) during fundamentals and health assessment courses. This change enabled students to apply clinical judgment and skills learned in the classroom to clinical practice and develop confidence. Finally, a collaborative virtual simulation by Weideman et al. (2016) strengthened the cultural competence of 136 ABSN students enrolled in two geographically distant schools. Technology enabled students to learn different perspectives about prenatal care by interacting with women from two culturally diverse local communities. Outcomes revealed significant increases in students' transcultural self-efficacy and plans of care.

Program Outcomes: Recruitment, Retention, and Predictors of Success

The rapid pace and intensive study involved in ABSN programs demand attention to recruiting diverse applicants who can successfully complete program requirements in a timely manner, pass their licensure examination on the first attempt, and successfully transition into clinical practice. Collecting and analyzing program outcome data from key stakeholders such as the graduates, employers, and faculty help determine program effectiveness and foster continuous quality improvement (Commission on Collegiate Nursing Education [CCNE], 2018).

A unique approach program was reported by Lee and Song (2021) who applied Kirkpatrick's four-level evaluation model (Kirkpatrick & Kirkpatrick, 2016) in their scoping review of educational outcomes for 15 ABSN and five AMSN programs. Results revealed strong evidence of graduates' academic achievements, employment rates, and program satisfaction but graduates felt challenged in being prepared for clinical and transitioning to their professional roles. Administrators of ABSN programs are urged to investigate the long-term impact of their programs and graduates on patient outcomes, employment settings, and the nursing workforce.

In an effort to increase workforce diversity within one school of nursing, Lewis et al. (2021) studied the outcomes after implementing a holistic admissions process in their 16-month ABSN program. This protocol considered non-academic data such as personal essays, demographics, and congruence with the mission. Comparisons between three applicant groups before and after the holistic process revealed that the new approach increased student diversity, sustained graduation and licensure pass rates, and decreased student remediation needs.

Transition to Clinical Practice

ABSN programs require careful follow-up after graduation to evaluate the performance of graduates in their new professional roles. Prior research often focused on the perspectives of key stakeholders such as employers, ABSN graduates, and faculty and compared these outcomes with graduates from traditional BSN programs during the immediate postgraduation period. Searching for evidence describing the experiences of ABSN graduates beyond their experiences as students or brand-new graduates, Schwartz and Gambescia (2017) conducted a literature review of past research. Surprisingly, results revealed only two dated studies (2013 and 2015).

In the same year, Brandt et al. (2017) captured the personal perspectives of seven ABSN graduates 12 to 15 months after graduation. Using qualitative interviews, the researchers asked the graduates to share their experiences in transitioning to clinical practice. Analysis revealed 11 themes that described the stress and intensity of clinical practice; importance of patient safety; fears related to being on their own; and how their fast-paced ABSN program prepared them for practice. Results mirrored the experiences of traditional four-year graduates and suggest postorientation support to develop the nurses' confidence.

Most recently, another qualitative approach was conducted by Hennessy (2018) to understand the transition to practice experiences of 12 graduates from five different ABSN programs across the southwestern US. Unlike previous transition studies, these nurses had been employed in clinical practice for at least two years. The authors reported that these ABSN alumni were socialized into the nursing profession, felt satisfied, and planned to stay in nursing.

NURSE PRACTITIONER PROGRAMS

Nurse practitioners (NP) comprise a robust growth component of the health care workforce with over 325,000 NPs licensed in the US in 2021 (American Association of Nurse Practitioners [AANP], 2021). The demand for nurse practitioner education continues to grow with 505 programs offering NP education as of 2021—406 master's level, 344 post-master's, and 258 DNP level programs (AACN, 2021b). The demand for APRNs (nurse practitioners, nurse anesthetists, and nurse midwives) is projected to increase over 45% from 2020 to 2030, a growth rate significantly higher than for other professions (Bureau of Labor Statistics, 2021).

Standards governing NP education include those relevant to all APRN roles established by professional organizations and accrediting bodies, as well as standards specific to the NP role such as those explicated in the *Criteria for Quality Nurse Practitioner Education Programs* document (National Task Force on Quality Nurse Practitioner Education, 2016). Programs preparing NPs also must comply with the expectations and requirements of the APRN Consensus Model (APRN Consensus Work Group and National Council of State Boards of Nursing APRN Advisory Committee, 2008).

Issues in the Clinical Education of NPs

Numerous challenges confront schools of nursing preparing NPs today. The most serious of these, with the potential to negatively impact programmatic outcomes, is a national shortage of qualified nursing faculty to meet enrollment demands, burgeoning student numbers, and growth in numbers of programs preparing NPs, which frequently leads to competition among schools for preceptors and quality clinical sites. Citing threats to patient safety, the American Medical Association (AMA) and some state medical associations continue to challenge the scope of practice expansions for NPs, often referencing what they perceive as inadequate academic and clinical preparation of NP students (AMA, 2021).

The current model of clinical education for NPs has traditionally been an apprenticeship model with one preceptor overseeing the clinical performance of one student at a time. This model is rapidly becoming unsustainable; as program and student numbers continue to increase, the expectations associated with NP and MD roles in practice become increasingly more complex, and increased scrutiny of NP program graduates' competence is being observed.

Alternative models of APRN clinical education, including competency-based education (CBE), are becoming increasingly prevalent and gaining momentum. There are numerous and varied competency standards and expectations of NP students and NP programs preparing competent graduates able to meet the demands of advanced clinical practice. Competency can be observed, measured, and assessed by an evaluator to determine achievement. Competency-based education has been in existence for more than six decades with multiple models, frameworks, and integration approaches described in the literature. Gruppen et al. (2016) described four essential components of CBE: (1) emphasis on expected and achieved outcomes, (2) focus on learner abilities, (3) decrease in time-based teaching and learning, and (4) facilitation of learner-centeredness. Challenges to the CBE approach include the definition, observation, and measurement of acquisition of competency (Hodges et al., 2019). Another challenge in NP education is the existence of significant expected levels of achievement, or milestones, related to clinical skill development before competency is assured (Anthamatten et al., 2020).

As of early 2022, no nationally standardized processes exist to assess competence of NP students. Moore and Hawkins-Walsh (2020) proposed the use of entrustable professional activities (EPAs) as a framework to translate competencies into clinical practice, comparable to what has been implemented in other health professions, by which NP student clinical competence can be assessed. The authors mapped six EPAs to NP core competencies which were then used by faculty to design eight clinically based scenarios to assess family nurse practitioner (FNP) student simulated clinical performance during an on-campus residency. Performance was assessed using EPA-based rubrics and checklists also designed by faculty. Each simulated clinical scenario was designed to assess one or two EPAs. Once student clinical rotations were completed, faculty assigned a utility score to each EPA grading rubric description. Study authors concluded EPA-based grading rubrics show potential utility as a competency-based measurement of assessing NP student clinical performance and may also be useful to faculty and administrators in identifying curricular gaps.

Clinical education and evaluation models, which have been tested and validated in other health care professions, illustrate some potentially feasible alternatives to traditional methods of clinical education and evaluation for NPs. For example, most accredited physical therapy (PT) educational programs in the US and Canada voluntarily use standardized competencies and competency-based clinical assessments developed in collaboration with the American Physical Therapy Association (Roach et al., 2012).

Several issues impact programs providing NP education: proliferation of mandated student assessment requirements, increased competition for clinical sites, and growing litigation and academic grievances related to lack of standardization in student assessment and evaluation practices. These concerns provide an impetus for the creation of NP competency development and validation, competency descriptors, and standardized clinical evaluation instruments.

NURSE ANESTHETIST PROGRAMS

Nurse anesthesia (NA) education in the US is over 100 years old and as of 2022, there were 128 accredited NA programs in the US and Puerto Rico (Council on Accreditation of Nurse Anesthesia Educational Programs [COA], 2021). The accreditation process for NA programs began in the early 1950s. The Council on Accreditation of Nurse Anesthesia Programs (COA) is the accrediting body for NA programs at the post-master's certificate, master's, and doctoral degree levels (COA, 2021). Beginning January 1, 2022, all students accepted into an accredited NA program must graduate with a doctoral degree as COA will no longer accredit programs offering the master's degree. Currently, 113 NA programs have been approved to award the doctoral credential as entry into practice.

One of the COA accreditation criteria under the Program of Study standard relates to student admission criteria. While the COA criteria delineate only two admission criteria, (1) registration as an RN (baccalaureate prepared) and (2) at least one year of experience as an RN in a critical care area, many NA programs use other admission criteria. An issue of particular relevance in program evaluation of NA programs includes analysis of student admission criteria and the impact of those criteria on student progression.

Student Admission and Progression

Admission into NA programs is a highly competitive process. Typical admission criteria include assessment of the applicant's overall grade point average (GPA), GPA in science courses, scores on the Graduate Record Examination (GRE), and years of acute care experience, especially in critical care areas. However, what is the state of the evidence linking admission criteria, other than those required by the COA, to the NA applicant's ability to successfully integrate theory and practice, which results in positive progression to graduation?

Ortega et al. (2013) conducted a systematic review to examine the evidence for evaluating applicants for admission into NA programs. Because of the limited number of sources and the weak and dated available evidence, the authors determined there were no consensus factors that predict overall student success in NA programs. However, admission criteria with predictive value for success in the anesthesia program included overall, science courses, and nursing program GPA. GRE scores were found to be less predictive in the studies reviewed. Similarly, in a study of four accredited NA programs to determine the validity of clinical evaluation tools, preadmission overall GPA was found to have high predictive value in determining students' abilities to transfer didactic knowledge to the clinical setting, troubleshoot equipment, and perform technical skills related to practice, thus suggesting that overall GPA is an important preadmission criterion to retain in NA programs (Collins & Callahan, 2014). The results of research examining and evaluating the utility of admission criteria factors lead to a growing body of evidence related to establishing research-based admission selection criteria for NA programs, which provides significant predictive value for student progression to graduation.

Student progression in NA programs is highly dependent on student clinical performance. The role of the clinical educator in NA programs is to assess and evaluate the daily clinical performance of student registered nurse anesthetists (SRNAs). Historically, there has been a lack of standardization and consistency in SRNA evaluation as competency-based clinical evaluation tools have not been validated or standardized. To address this deficit, in 2016 the COA Board created the Common Clinical Assessment Tool (CCAT) Special Interest Group. The charge of the group was to develop a standardized clinical evaluation instrument. Elisha et al. (2020) described the process for development of the CCAT, which included the use of the Delphi method to determine competencies, competency descriptors, and progression indicators. As of this writing, the use of the tool is optional, and analysis and evaluation of the tool by clinical educators is ongoing. Adoption of a standardized evaluation instrument in SRNA education is important for clinical evaluation consistency and reliability in and among CRNA programs; a tool would also enable program administrators to implement relevant programmatic changes in compliance with accreditation standards, and is an important step forward in competency-based assessment and evaluation of SRNAs (Elisha et al., 2020).

DOCTORAL PROGRAMS IN NURSING

Doctor of Nursing Practice and Doctor of Philosophy/Nursing Science

The IOM's (2010) goal of doubling the number of doctorally prepared nurses by 2020 in an effort to alleviate the shortage of nurses prepared to address the nation's current and future health care needs was attained, as evidenced by the exponential growth of individuals awarded nursing doctoral degrees (DNP/PhD) from 1,184 graduates in 2010 to 9,917 graduates in 2020 (Future of Nursing Campaign for Action, 2021b). Data also reflect increased numbers of graduates from unrepresented racial/ethnic minorities from 2011 to 2020 in PhD (19.6% to 28%) and DNP programs (17.1% to 36.7%) (AACN, 2021b). In 2019–2020, males comprised 11.4% of research-focused and 12.6% of DNP program graduates (AACN, 2021b).

Both practice- and research-focused doctoral programs are essential for meeting the nation's health care needs by advancing nursing practice and nursing science. In addition to the traditional post-master's pathway to these doctorates, several institutions have designed innovative programs in which nurses can earn their doctoral degrees in a more streamlined and timely manner, such as DNP to PhD programs that facilitate DNP graduates attaining their PhD (AACN, 2021b). Loescher et al. (2021) describe successful outcomes of their decade-old dual doctoral nursing degree that blends advanced practice and nursing science. According to the authors, their dual program is one of five such programs offered by major universities in the US.

Some schools of nursing offer programs that support baccalaureate-prepared nurses to earn their doctoral degrees early in their professional careers. Greene et al. (2017) describe a clinical nurse fellowship targeted to students enrolled in BSN-PhD programs in three schools of nursing in collaboration with their health system partners. Among its many benefits, this fellowship helped students integrate clinical practice with classroom learning and develop scholarship through research and nursing practice innovations.

Several schools with DNP programs have developed academic-practice partnerships that build upon the strengths and resources of all stakeholders (Hartjes et al., 2021; Hinch et al., 2020; Melander et al., 2021; Vessey et al., 2021). Reynolds and colleagues (2021) outline the positive outcomes of a school's unique collaboration that resulted in a one-year DNP postdoctoral program aimed to strengthen competencies in quality improvement and nursing science.

Because practice- and research-focused doctoral programs prepare graduates for different, yet complementary roles, they require diverse program elements, resources, and evaluation. The AACN has outlined these differences based on program objectives, programs of study, student career interests, faculty, resources, and program outcomes (AACN, 2014).

Practice-Focused Doctorate in Nursing: DNP

As a practice-focused doctorate, the DNP prepares advanced practice nurses to "improve patient outcomes and translate research into practice" (AACN, 2014, p.1). The DNP was proposed as the terminal degree for advanced practice nurses including NPs, clinical nurse specialists, certified nurse-midwives, certified registered nurse anesthetists, and others with an interest to "implement the science developed by nurse researchers" (AACN, 2015, p.1).

As of October 2020, there were 357 DNP programs in 50 US states and the District of Columbia, with 106 programs in progress (AACN, 2020a). Over the past decade, DNP programs have more than doubled with steady increases each year, from 182 programs in 2011 to 386 programs in 2020 (AACN, 2021b). Growth in DNP student enrollments have also been robust, with 8,973 students in 2011 to 39,530 in 2020 (AACN, 2021b); graduations increased from 7,039 to 7,944 during 2019 to 2020 (AACN, 2020a).

Research-Focused Doctorates: PhD and DNS

The PhD and doctor of nursing science (DNS) degrees are research-focused doctorates that "prepare nurses at the highest level of nursing science to conduct research to advance the science of nursing" (AACN, 2014, p.1). Until recently, the *Research Focused Doctoral Program in Nursing: Pathways to Excellence* guided research-focused doctoral programs (AACN, 2010). An updated version is currently under review and offers a "vision" focused on doctoral students, faculty, and curriculum and evaluation (AACN, 2021c).

Over the past decade, the growth in new PhD programs has been much slower than the trends reported for DNP programs, with 126 PhD programs in 2011 increasing to 147 programs in 2020 (AACN, 2021b). In fact, enrollment actually decreased over the same decade by nearly 15% from 4,907 to 4,626 students (AACN, 2021b). From 2016 to 2020, student enrollments decreased by 5.9% and graduations decreased by 2.2% (AACN, 2021b)

Evolving changes in doctoral education demands ongoing assessment and systematic evaluation. Particular attention should be given to: (1) faculty numbers and qualifications, (2) curriculum and role-specific competencies, and (3) program outcomes.

Faculty Numbers and Qualifications

Doctoral programs must have a sufficient number of faculty who are qualified to meet the needs of the nursing program (CCNE, 2018). Nursing programs cited shortages of faculty and clinical sites among the primary reasons for not offering admission to 8,471 qualified master's and 3,157 doctoral applicants (AACN, 2020b). Nearly 90% of vacant faculty positions require or prefer a doctoral degree. While multiple strategies are currently in place to address this shortage, master's and doctoral programs have not been able to meet the rising demand for potential faculty (AACN, 2020b).

Since faculty qualifications differ for teaching in the two types of doctoral programs, attention needs to be given to faculty development. Lazear and Hemphill (2020) shared promising outcomes related to their piloted faculty development program aimed to increase the confidence of eight doctoral-prepared faculty members in two affiliated schools of nursing. The intervention was based on the faculty's self-identified learning needs and delivered through didactic and experiential activities with mentoring. Results revealed significant increases in faculty's confidence levels, particularly in topics such as DNP project analysis and dissemination.

Curriculum Content and Competencies

Since DNP and PhD/DNS programs prepare nurse leaders for two complementary yet different roles, faculty must design role-specific curricula and obtain resources, such as clinical sites and preceptors, that will enable graduates to develop their expected roles. New curriculum standards for the DNP degree that are outlined in the recently endorsed *The Essentials: Core Competencies for Professional Nursing Education,* give attention to advanced-level competencies and sub-competencies organized by ten domains (AACN, 2021d). This new model emphasizes a competency-based approach with required DNP scholarly projects that "improve clinical practice" (AACN, 2021d, p.24). As previously mentioned, a newly revised *Research Focused Doctoral Program in Nursing: Pathways to Excellence* provides schools with guidance to advance nursing science (AACN, 2021c).

Advancements in curriculum standards and competencies provide opportunities for developing creative teaching-learning practices. Howard et al. (2020) implemented a novel teaching model in collaboration with their clinical affiliate in which both faculty and DNP-prepared affiliate clinical leaders taught DNP courses. Results revealed several short-term benefits related to stakeholder satisfaction and program outcomes.

Program Outcomes

DNP programs are accredited by the CCNE (2018) or the Commission for Nursing Education Accreditation (CNEA) (2021); however, PhD/DNS programs follow institutional policies regarding external review (AACN, 2021c). Administrators of doctoral programs should conduct ongoing and systematic program evaluations based on doctoral-specific roles. Evidence collected from various stakeholders should be incorporated as ongoing quality improvement.

Turkson-Ocran et al. (2020) illustrate the value of program evaluation in their comprehensive review of 191 DNP projects completed over a decade at their institution. Results included aggregate data that described targeted participants, settings, designs, dissemination, and overall themes. This information provided opportunities for "transformative changes in advanced practice" (Turkson-Ocran et al., 2020, p. 4090). Using a similar strategy, Samldone et al. (2019) reviewed 113 PhD dissertations completed at their school over the past decade and compared outcomes based on the use of traditional versus alternate dissertation formats. Graduates who used alternate dissertation formats had more favorable dissemination outcomes (numbers and timeliness of publications) compared to their colleagues who used the traditional format.

Summary

This chapter has presented the latest evidence-based research on program assessment and evaluation pertinent to RN to BSN, accelerated second career programs, nurse practitioner, nurse anesthesia, and doctoral programs in nursing. Program administrators and faculty charged with program evaluation responsibilities can incorporate this information in the design of assessment and evaluation processes in support of continual program and performance improvement.

References

American Association of Colleges of Nursing. (2008). *The essentials of baccalaureate education for professional nursing practice.* https://www.aacnnursing.org/Portals/42/Publications/BaccEssentials08.pdf

American Association of Colleges of Nursing. (2010). *The research-focused doctoral program in nursing: Pathways to excellence.* www.aacn.nche.edu/education-resources/PhDTaskForceReport.pdf

American Association of Colleges of Nursing. (2014). *Key differences between DNP and PhD/DNS Programs.* https://www.aacnnursing.org/Portals/42/DNP/ContrastGrid.pdf

American Association of Colleges of Nursing. (2015). *The doctor of nursing practice: Current*

issues and clarifying recommendations.
https://www.pncb.org/sites/default/files/
2017-02/AACN_DNP_Recommendations.pdf

American Association of Colleges of Nursing.
(2019). *Fact sheet: Accelerated baccalaureate and master's degrees in nursing.*
https://www.aacnnursing.org/News-
Information/Fact-Sheets/Accelerated-
Programs

American Association of Colleges of Nursing.
(2020a). *Fact sheet: The doctor of nursing practice (DNP).* https://www.aacnnursing.
org/Portals/42/News/Factsheets/DNP-
Factsheet.pdf

American Association of Colleges of Nursing.
(2020b). *Nursing faculty shortage fact sheet.*
https://www.aacnnursing.org/Portals/
42/News/Factsheets/Faculty-Shortage-
Factsheet.pdf

American Association of Colleges of Nursing
(2021a). *Student enrollment surged in U.S.
schools of nursing in 2020 despite challenges presented by the pandemic.*
https://www.aacnnursing.org/News-
Information/Press-Releases/View/ArticleId/
24802/2020-survey-data-student-enrollment

American Association of Colleges of Nursing
(2021b). *2020–2021 enrollment and graduations in baccalaureate and graduate programs in nursing.* American Association of
Colleges of Nursing.

American Association of Colleges of Nursing.
(2021c). *The research-focused doctoral
program in nursing: Pathways to excellence.*
https://www.aacnnursing.org/Portals/42/
News/Position-Statements/DRAFT-
Research-Focused-Doctoral-Pathways-
to-Excellence.pdf

American Association of Colleges of Nursing.
(2021d). *The essentials: Core competencies
for professional nursing education.*
https://www.aacnnursing.org/Portals/42/
AcademicNursing/pdf/Essentials-2021.pdf

American Association of Nurse Practitioners.
(2021). *NP fact sheet.* https://aanp.org/
about/all-about-nps/np-fact-sheet

American Medical Association. (2021). *AMA
successfully fights scope of practice
expansions that threaten patient safety.*
https://ama-assn.org/practice-management/

scope-practice/ama-sucessfully-fights-
scope-practice-expansion-threaten

Anthamatten, A., Pfieffer, M. L., Richmond,
A., & Glassford, M. (2020). Exploring the
utility of entrustable professional activities as a framework to enhance nurse
practitioner education. *Nurse Educator,
45*(2), 83–87. https://doi.org/10.1097/
NNE.0000000000000697

APRN Consensus Work Group and National
Council of State Boards of Nursing APRN
Advisory Committee. (2008). *Consensus
model for APRN regulation: Licensure,
accreditation, certification, and education.*
http://www.aacn.nche.edu/education-
resources/APRNReport.pdf

Baxter, K. (2018). Curriculum planning for
undergraduate nursing programs. In S. B.
Keating & S. S. DeBoor (Eds.), *Curriculum
development and evaluation in nursing*
(4th ed., pp. 123–145). Springer.

Brandt, C. L., Boellaard, M. R., & Wilberding,
K. M. (2017). Accelerated second-degree
bachelor of science in nursing graduates'
transition to professional practice. *Journal
of Continuing Education in Nursing, 48*(1),
14–19. https://doi.org/10.3928/00220124-
20170110-05

Bureau of Labor Statistics. (2021). *Occupational
outlook handbook: Nurse anesthetists, nurse
midwives, and nurse practitioner.* Retrieved
January 29, 2022, from www.bls.gov/ooh/
healthcare/nurse-anesthetists-nurse-
midwives-and-nurse-practitioners.htm

Burgess, A., & Medina-Smuck, M. (2018).
Collaborative testing using quizzes as a
method to improve undergraduate nursing student engagement and interaction.
Nursing Education Perspectives, 39(3),
178–179. https://doi.org/10.1097/01.
NEP.0000000000000223

Christoffersen, J. E. (2017). Teaching accelerated second-degree nursing students:
Educators from across the United States
share their wisdom. *Nursing Forum, 52*(2),
111–117. https://doi.org/10.1111/nuf.12174

Cipher, D. J., Mancini, M. E., & Shrestha, S.
(2017). Predictors of persistence and
success in an accelerated online RN to
BSN program. *Journal of Nursing Education,*

56(9), 522–526. https://doi.org/10.3928/01484834-20170817-02

Collins, S., & Callahan, M. F. (2014). A call for change: Clinical evaluation of student registered nurse anesthetists. *AANA Journal, 82*(1), 65–72.

Commission on Collegiate Nursing Education. (2018). *Standards for accreditation of baccalaureate and graduate nursing programs (Amended 2018)*. https://www.aacnnursing.org/Portals/42/CCNE/PDF/Standards-Final-2018.pdf

Commission for Nursing Education Accreditation. (2021). *Accreditation standards for nursing education programs*. https://irp.cdn-website.com/cc12ee87/files/uploaded/CNEA%20Standards%20October%202021.pdf\

Council on Accreditation of Nurse Anesthesia Educational Programs. (2021). *Accreditation*. http://home.coa.us.com/accreditation/Pages/default.aspx

Elisha, S., Bonanno, L., Porche, D., Mercante, D.E., & Gerbasi, F. (2020). Development of a common clinical evaluation in nurse anesthesia evaluation. *AANA Journal, 88*(1), 11–17.

Future of Nursing Campaign for Action. (2021a). *Welcome to the future of nursing: Campaign for action dashboard*. Retrieved January 29, 2022, from https://campaignforaction.org/wp-content/uploads/2021/02/Dashboard-Indicator-Updates_Fall-2021.pdf

Future of Nursing Campaign for Action. (2021b). *Number of people receiving nursing doctoral degrees annually*. Retrieved January 29, 2022 from https://campaignforaction.org/resource/number-people-receiving-nursing-doctoral-degrees-annually/

Greene, M. Z., FitzPatrick, M. K., Romano, J., Aiken, L. H., & Richmond, T. S. (2017). Clinical fellowship for an innovative, integrated BSN-PhD program: An academic and practice partnership. *Journal of Professional Nursing, 33*(4), 282–286. https://doi.org/10.1016/j.profnurs.2016.12.001

Gruppen, L. D., Burkhardt, J. C., Fitzgerald, J. T., Funnell, M., Haftel, H. M., Lypson, M. L., Mullan, P. B., Santen, S. A., Sheets, K. J., Stalburg, C. M., & Vasquez, J. A. (2016). Competency-based education: programme design and challenges to implementation.

Medical Education, 50(5), 532–539. https://doi.org/10.1111/medu.12977

Harlan, M. D., Beach, M., & Blazeck, A. (2021). Preparing ABSN students for early entry and success in the clinical setting: Flipping both class and skills lab with the Socratic method. *International Journal of Nursing Education Scholarship, 18*(1), 10.1515/ijnes-2021-0044. https://doi.org/10.1515/ijnes-2021-0044

Hartjes, T. M., Starr, K., Kittelson, S., & Duckworth, L. (2021). Navigating the doctor of nursing practice project within an academic practice partnership. *Journal of the American Association of Nurse Practitioners, 33*(12), 1125–1130. https://doi.org/10.1097/JXX.0000000000000600

Hennessy, L. (2018). The lived experience of registered nurses educated in accelerated second-degree bachelor of science in nursing programs: A hermeneutic phenomenological research study. *Nurse Education in Practice, 28*, 264–269. https://doi.org/10.1016/j.nepr.2017.09.010

Hinch, B. K., Livesay, S., Stifter, J., & Brown, F. Jr. (2020). Academic-practice partnerships: Building a sustainable model for doctor of nursing practice (DNP) projects. *Journal of Professional Nursing, 36*(6), 569–578. https://doi.org/10.1016/j.profnurs.2020.08.008

Hodges, A. L., Konicki, A. J., Talley, M. H., Bordelon, C. J., Holland, A. C., & Galin, F. S. (2019). Competency-based education in transitioning nurse practitioner students from education into practice. *Journal of the American Association of Nurse Practitioners, 31*(11), 675–682. https://doi.org/10.1097/JXX.0000000000000327

Hooper, J. I., McEwen, M., & Mancini, M. (2013). A regulatory challenge: Creating a metric for quality RN to BSN programs. *Journal of Nursing Regulation, 4*(2), 34–38. https://doi.org/10.1016/S2155-8356(15)30156-3

Howard, P. B., Williams, T. E., El-Mallakh, P., Melander, S., Tharp-Barrie, K., Lock, S., & MacCallum, T. (2020). An innovative teaching model in an academic-practice partnership for a doctor of nursing practice program. *Journal of Professional Nursing,*

36(5), 285–291. https://doi.org/10.1016/j.profnurs.2020.04.010

Institute of Medicine. (2010). The future of nursing: Leading change, advancing health. http://www.iom.edu/Reports/2010/The-Future-of-Nursing-Leading-Change-Advancing-Health.aspx

Jacobs, A. (2021). "Nursing is in crisis": Staff shortages put patients at risk. Retrieved January 29, 2022, from https://www.nytimes.com/2021/08/21/health/covid-nursing-shortage-delta.html

Kirkpatrick, J. D., & Kirkpatrick, W. K. (2016). *Kirkpatrick's four levels of training evaluation*. ATD Press.

Lazear, J., & Hemphill, J. C. (2020). Preparing faculty to lead doctor of nursing practice projects: A faculty development pilot project. *Journal of Professional Nursing, 36*(6), 673–680. https://doi.org/10.1016/j.profnurs.2020.09.009

Lee, H., & Song, Y. (2021). Kirkpatrick model evaluation of accelerated second-degree nursing programs: A scoping review. *The Journal of Nursing Education, 60*(5), 265–271. https://doi.org/10.3928/01484834-20210420-05

Lewis, L., Biederman, D., Hatch, D., Li, A., Turner, K., & Molloy, M. A. (2021). Outcomes of a holistic admissions process in an accelerated baccalaureate nursing program. *Journal of Professional Nursing, 37*(4), 714–720. https://doi.org/10.1016/j.profnurs.2021.05.006

Linton, M., Knecht, L., Dabney, B., & Koonmen, J. (2019). Student-centered curricular revisions to facilitate transition from associate degree in nursing bachelor of science in nursing education. *Teaching and Learning in Nursing, 14,* 279–822. https://doi.org/10.1016/j.teln.2019.06.008

Loescher, L. J., Love, R., & Badger, T. (2021). Breaking new ground? The dual (PhD-DNP) doctoral degree in nursing. *Journal of Professional Nursing, 37*(2), 429–434. https://doi.org/10.1016/j.profnurs.2020.05.001

Matthews, M. B., & Travis, L. L. (1994). Research on the baccalaureate completion process for RNs. *Annual Review of Nursing Research, 12,* 149–171. https://doi:10.1891/0739-6686.12.1.149

McElwain, S. D., Rhodes, K. A., Carr, K. L., & Lawrence, M. C. (2021). Early immersion clinical for an accelerated BSN nursing program. *Nursing Education Perspectives, 42*(6), E107–E108. https://doi.org/10.1097/01.NEP.0000000000000675

McEwen, M., White, M. J., Pullis, B. R., & Krawtz, S. (2014). Essential content in RN-BSN programs. *Journal of Professional Nursing, 30*(4), 333–340. https://doi.org/10.1016/j.profnurs.2013.10.003

Melander, S., Hampton, D., Garritano, N., Makowski, A., Hardin-Pierce, M., Scott, L., Tovar, E., & Biddle, M. (2021). Strengthening the impact of doctor of nursing practice projects in education and clinical practice. *The Nurse Practitioner, 46*(8), 33–38. https://doi.org/10.1097/01.NPR.0000751804.78165.5a

Moore, J., & Hawkins-Walsh, E. (2020). Evaluating nurse practitioner student competencies: Application of entrustable professional activities. *Journal of Nursing Education, 59*(12). https://doi.org/10.3928/01484834-20201118-11

National Task Force on Quality Nurse Practitioner Education. (2016). *Criteria for evaluation of nurse practitioner programs* (5th ed.). National Organization of Nurse Practitioner Faculties. https://cdn.ymaws.com/www.nonpf.org/resource/resmgr/Docs/EvalCriteria2016Final.pdf

O'Brien, B., & Renner, A. (2000). Nurses online: Career mobility for registered nurses. *Journal of Professional Nursing, 16*(1), 13–20. https://doi.org/10.1016/s8755-7223(00)80007-1

Ortega, K. H., Burns, S. M., Hussey, L. C., Schmidt, J., & Austin, P. N. (2013). Predicting success in nurse anesthesia programs: An evidence-based review of admission criteria. *AANA Journal, 81*(3), 183–189.

Perfetto, L. M. (2019). Preparing the nurse of the future: Emergent themes in online RN-BSN education. *Nursing Education Perspectives, 40*(1), 18–24. https://doi.org/10.1097/01.NEP.0000000000000378

Reynolds, S. S., Howard, V., Uzarski, D., Granger, B. B., Fuchs, M. A., Mason, L., & Broome, M. E. (2021). An innovative DNP post-doctorate program to improve quality improvement and implementation science skills. *Journal of Professional Nursing, 37*(1), 48–52. https://doi.org/10.1016/j.profnurs.2020.12.005

Roach, K. E., Frost, J. S., Francis, N. J., Giles, S., & Nordrum, A. D. (2012), Validation of the revised physical therapist clinical performance instrument (PT CPI): Version 2006. *Physical Therapy, 92*(3), 416–428. https://doi.org/10.2522/ptj.20110129

Robertson, S., Canary, C. W., Orr, M., Herberg, P., & Rutledge, D. N. (2010). Factors related to progression and graduation rates for RN to bachelor of science in nursing programs: Searching for realistic benchmarks. *Journal of Professional Nursing, 26*(2), 99–107. https://doi.org/10.1016/j.profnurs.2009.09.003

Schwartz, J., & Gambescia, S. F. (2017). A literature review of research on what has become of accelerated second-degree baccalaureate nursing graduates. *Nursing Education Perspectives, 38*(1), 29–31. https://doi.org/10.1097/01.NEP.0000000000000100

Shatto, B., L'Ecuyer, K., & Quinn, J. (2017). Retention of content utilizing a flipped classroom approach. *Nursing Education Perspectives, 38*(4), 206–208. https://doi.org/10.1097/01.NEP.0000000000000138

Sitzman, K., Carpenter, T., & Cherry, K. (2020). Student perceptions related to immediate workplace usefulness of RN to BSN

program content. *Nurse Educator, 45*(5), 5, 265–268. https://doi.org/10.1097/NNE.0000000000000775

Stokowski, L. A. (2011). Overhauling nursing education. *Medscape Nurses News.* Retrieved from http://www.medscape.com/viewarticle/736236

Turkson-Ocran, R. N., Spaulding, E. M., Renda, S., Pandian, V., Rittler, H., Davidson, P. M., Nolan, M. T., & D'Aoust, R. (2020). A 10-year evaluation of projects in a doctor of nursing practice programme. *Journal of Clinical Nursing, 29*(21–22), 4090–4103. https://doi.org/10.1111/jocn.15435

Vessey, J. A., Wentzell, K., Wendt, J., & Glynn, D. (2021). DNP scholarly projects: Unintended consequences for academic-practice partnerships. *Journal of Professional Nursing, 37*(3), 516–520. https://doi.org/10.1016/j.profnurs.2021.03.007

Wagner, J., Foster, B., & O'Sullivan, R. (2020). Measuring learning outcomes in a RN to BSN program. *Teaching and Learning in Nursing, 15,* 19–24. https://doi.org/10.1016/j.teln.2019.07.006

Weideman, Y. L., Young, L., Lockhart, J. S., Grund, F. J., Fridline, M. M., & Panas, M. (2016). Strengthening cultural competence in prenatal care with a virtual community: Building capacity through collaboration. *Journal of Professional Nursing, 32*(5S), S48–S53. https://doi.org/10.1016/j.profnurs.2016.03.004.

10

Evaluation and Accreditation of Health Care Simulation Programs

Kim Leighton, PhD, RN, CHSE, CHSOS, FSSH, FAAN, ANEF

Nicole Petsas Blodgett, PhD, RN, CHSE

Simulation, as a teaching strategy, is ubiquitous in nursing education, being integrated to various levels throughout all types of nursing education including nursing and patient care assistants, licensed practical or vocational nursing, and associate and baccalaureate programs. Simulation is used as an adjunct for advanced practice registered nurse (APRN) programs, and master's degree nursing education students learn how to integrate simulation into their future courses. Research studies and projects assessing outcomes related to simulation training are often found within Doctor of Philosophy (PhD) and Doctor of Nursing Practice (DNP) programs but are now becoming their own entity as we see the rise of degrees dedicated to health care simulation.

Traditional clinical experiences involving face-to-face interactions between students and patients have historically been the gold standard for the application of knowledge in health professions education. However, emerging evidence has revealed that traditional clinical experiences may not be as effective as once believed due to lack of documented outcomes data in the research literature (Leighton et al., 2021; Leighton et al., 2022). A substantial body of evidence shows that high-quality simulation-based experiences lead to similar or better learning outcomes than traditional clinical experiences. For example, the National Council of State Boards of Nursing (NCSBN) (Hayden et al., 2014) reported findings from a multisite longitudinal study that supported simulation as a replacement for up to 50% of traditional clinical hours in undergraduate nursing education under certain specific conditions. Almost immediately, the NCSBN followed with guidelines designed to help boards of nursing evaluate the use of simulation when used as a substitute for traditional clinical and to support the development of an evidence-based undergraduate nursing curriculum that included simulation (Alexander et al., 2015). Heavy emphasis was placed on proving that simulation was being conducted at a high enough standard to warrant replacing traditional clinical hours. As simulation also carried the heavy price tag of high-tech equipment, small learning groups, supplies, new or refurbished space, faculty development, and ongoing warranty and maintenance costs, it was also held to a high standard of proof of efficiency and effectiveness. Essentially, it was vital to evaluate the outcomes of simulation to prove its worth. A variety of instruments and methods of evaluation have been developed in the past decade to not only support the use of simulation, but to assist faculty and simulationists to improve their practice, learning outcomes, curricular integration, and operational efficiencies.

This chapter provides a brief history of the growth of simulation in nursing programs with a general overview of the major types and purposes of simulation in nursing education. Three types of evaluation (formative, summative, and high-stakes) are reviewed, and various data collection methods are presented with their challenges and strengths. Numerous constructs related to simulation can be evaluated, and the reader is presented with an overview of the categories of evaluation instruments and commentary on how to best align the instruments with the learning objectives and level of the learners. Following a discussion on reliability and validity, and special considerations related to high-stakes assessment, the reader is guided on how to locate evaluation instruments aligned with their evaluation needs. The second half of the chapter focuses on the accreditation process, whereby accreditation establishes that a simulation program has upheld the highest standards of simulation education and training. Examples of the types of accreditation, the associated benefits, and program activities leading up to accreditation are presented.

SIMULATION GROWTH IN ACADEMIC NURSING PROGRAMS

Simulation has existed in various formats in nursing programs for over a century. Many nurses will recall using oranges to learn how to give an injection, giving bed baths to one another, and even inserting intravenous (IV) needles and nasogastric tubes (NGT) into their peers in the skills lab. While oranges have stood the test of time, risk management, ethical considerations, and the rising availability of simulation models have led to decreased use of vulnerable people (the student) for the practice of skills. Simulation resources have been created that are durable, relatively inexpensive, and provide opportunities for repetitive practice that leads to mastery learning. These simulation products have evolved over the past two decades to move from task training to including full-body simulators, virtual reality, and the use of trained standardized or simulated participants (Leighton, 2017). A general overview of major types of simulation commonly used in nursing education, with examples and purposes for each type is provided in Table 10.1.

As Gaba (2004) famously said, "Simulation is a technique—not a technology—to replace or amplify real experiences with guided experiences that evoke or replicate substantial aspects of the real world in a fully interactive manner" (p. i2). This should have given pause to the many organizations that used donor money, grant funding, and large budgets to purchase simulation equipment, often in bulk. Forgotten in the purchase of the technology was the investment in training and education of those who would facilitate the implementation of this new teaching strategy. Often, the skills lab coordinator became assigned to manage manikin-based simulators because they had already been teaching with a variety of static task trainers (also a type of simulation). Initial adoption of manikin-based simulation was seen as an adjunct to the task trainers and logically added to existing skills lab work. However, it was not long before the potential power of manikin-based simulation to impact clinical judgment, clinical reasoning, prioritization, teamwork, communication, and other higher-order thinking skills became apparent. Simulation scenarios were touted as ways to practice patient care in an environment safe for the patient, one in which mistakes could be made, the outcomes of mistakes discussed in debriefing, and opportunities to

TABLE 10.1		
Major Types of Simulation		
Type of Simulation	**Examples**	**Purpose**
Task Trainers/ Procedural Simulators	IV, NGT, urinary catheter insertion models, wound care model	Repetitive practice of skills on durable equipment that withstands the repetition
Manikins/Patient Simulators	Full or partial body adult, pediatric, infant, newborn, premature, obstetrical, trauma	Create patient care situations to promote assessment, prioritization, communication, higher-order thinking skills
Standardized/ Simulated Patients and Participants (SP)	Person trained to portray symptoms and behaviors of a patient with abdominal pain; person trained to portray the role of an anxious family member	Provides opportunity for communication with the patient and others present in the scenario; often used for Objective Structured Clinical Exams with SP providing feedback to the learner
Hybrid	Wearable tracheostomy suction shirt or injection pad attached to a human (or manikin)	Allows the learner to practice the skill and communicate with a real person
Screen-based Simulation	Scenario delivered via Zoom with learners observing from home while instructor or students participate in person; program created for learners to respond to patient situations	Allows groups of learners to participate in scenarios when not in the same room; can be synchronous or asynchronous
Virtual Reality (VR)	Administer medications, insert urinary catheter, provide care to virtual patient	VR creates 3D space to provide spatial presence; may or may not require a headset

IV, intravenous; NGT, nasogastric tube.

redo the scenario could be provided. This type of teaching strategy, commonly referred to as simulation-based experiences (SBEs), was directly opposed to the premise of many nursing skills laboratories, where checklists were used to ensure the learner completed skills in correct steps using the precise method. The failure to complete the skill according to the checklist could result in consequences as high as the student being terminated from the nursing program. These two ways of teaching—clinical skills and simulation— challenged how we evaluated nursing students.

EVALUATION OF NURSING SIMULATION

Clinical skills activities and simulation scenarios are built from a needs assessment that considers one or more courses, program levels, clinical sites, or an entire curriculum to determine the learning gaps that can best be met in a simulation learning environment. The needs assessment drives the creation of learning objectives that form the basis of the entire simulation activity. Once learning objectives are created, educators should consider how they measure whether the learning objectives are met. Now is the time to think about evaluation. Many consider evaluation a last step in the process; however, the educator should plan ahead for how they will evaluate the learning outcomes of the activity.

Evaluation is the process of making judgments about learning, clinical performance, employee competence, and educational programs (Oermann & Gaberson, 2021). This definition supports the foundational need for nursing programs to have a comprehensive evaluation program for simulation that allows educators to make those judgments based on data. Simulation research tends to report siloed outcomes related to skill acquisition, debriefing, prebriefing, and performance, among others, but there remains minimal attention to creating a comprehensive evaluation program for simulation in nursing education (Leighton et al., 2020). The Healthcare Simulation Standards of Best Practice™ for Evaluation of Learning and Performance (International Nursing Association for Clinical Simulation and Learning [INACSL] Standards Committee, McMahon et al., 2021) stated that SBEs "support evaluation of the learner's knowledge, skills, attitudes, and behaviors demonstrated in the cognitive, psychomotor, and/or affective domains of learning" (p. 54). Evaluation is further differentiated as formative, summative, and high-stakes assessment (Table 10.2). Each type of evaluation is aligned with its purpose, and an example is provided for when the evaluation strategy may be implemented. It is important the student understands which type of evaluation will be conducted so they can prepare accordingly. The educator should use the correct type of evaluation instrument to align with the chosen evaluation.

TABLE 10.2

Types of Evaluation

Types of Evaluation	Purpose	Example
Formative	Facilitate learning, development Monitor, assist with progress toward goal Receive constructive feedback May be concurrent with instruction	Students are practicing how to don sterile gloves, while an instructor observes and points out when sterile technique is broken, followed by tips on how to avoid the same error next time.
Summative	May be at end of learning period Given feedback about the achievement according to criteria Process of determining competence; compared to a standard May be graded	At the end of the clinical course, the student receives a grade of B for simulation, with feedback that they did not consistently communicate with their simulated patient, ignoring the questions the patient asked. Communication was a criterion to meet on the evaluation instrument.
High-stakes	Outcome has major consequence Done at a discrete point in time	The advanced practice registered nurse student was terminated from the program when unable to correctly diagnose the simulated patient's presenting problem 30% of the time.

CHOOSING EVALUATION METHODS AND INSTRUMENTS

Evaluation data can be gathered using a variety of individual or combined methods to examine various constructs before, during, and after SBEs (Leighton et al., 2020). Construct refers to "any intangible attribute of a person, group of people, or system" (Santomauro et al., 2020, p. 342). Common constructs for SBE include attributes of the participant (i.e., competency, anxiety, communication) and the simulation experience (i.e., prebriefing, debriefing); however, the facilitator (i.e., performance scenario design) and operational aspects of the experience (i.e., room and equipment usage hours) should also be evaluated to create a comprehensive simulation program evaluation (Leighton et al., 2020). The constructs under evaluation need to align with the purpose (formative, summative, high-stakes) and learning objectives of the training, as well as the level of the learner (e.g., novice, proficient) (Table 10.3). While good evaluation is always important, the rigor must be raised when the evaluation is summative or high-stakes. The literature is replete with studies of various constructs related to simulation, many of which align with the Jeffries NLN Simulation Theory constructs (Jeffries, 2016).

TABLE 10.3				
Example Alignment of Evaluation Purpose, Learner Level, Learning Objectives, and Constructs for Evaluation				
Purpose	**Learner Level**	**Learning Objective**	**Constructs**	**Evaluation Method**
Formative	Novice, 1st year	During the cardiopulmonary arrest scenario, the student will demonstrate proper cardiopulmonary resuscitation technique	Competency Performance Knowledge Anxiety Technical skills	Dichotomous checklist Self-report measure
Summative	Advanced beginner, 2nd year	During the cardiopulmonary arrest scenario, the student will follow the order and timeline of the basic life support algorithm without deviation.	Competency Performance Communication Self-efficacy Technical skills	Simulator data collected on compression depth, speed, hand placement, time Dichotomous checklist Observation rubric
High-stakes	Teams of graduating students	During the cardiopulmonary arrest scenario, the students will work as a team following the basic life support algorithm without deviation	Teamwork Communication Higher order thinking skills Prioritization	Observation rubric with established interrater reliability Checklist of teamwork behaviors Determine if evaluating team or individual team members

Categories of Measurement

A variety of instruments and methods exist to evaluate the constructs related to simulation. Categories of measurement instruments include self-reporting, behavioral marker systems, and global rating scales of individuals, as well as teams (Santomauro et al., 2020). Evaluation data can also be obtained through feedback systems such as haptics and virtual reality analysis, as well as through reflective conversations, like those that occur in debriefing. Each has its own benefits and challenges related to ease of use, objective versus subjective data, and potential bias (Table 10.4).

Often, educators begin with an evaluation of satisfaction with the simulation experience. This is an example of a Level 1 Reaction on the New World Kirkpatrick Model (NWKM), which considers whether participants feel engaged, there is relevance to their jobs, and the training is favorable (Kirkpatrick & Kirkpatrick, 2016). These data are related to training effectiveness; however, it is not enough that learners are satisfied with their experience. The evaluation needs to be in more depth, although this type of data serves a purpose. When attempting to get stakeholders on board with simulation, whether they are faculty, other students, or even potential funders, it is helpful to share with them that learners enjoy learning with simulation. Perceptions are also commonly evaluated, but this also presents challenges. A common practice in simulation is to assign roles to the learners, but during debriefing, the educator often learns that students do not always agree on what happened. This occurs because each role observes from a different vantage point. The student assigned to assess the patient will not hear what another student is reporting on the phone or see what the medication nurse is preparing to administer. The student who is documenting may have the best overall perception and understanding, as will any observers. Using perceptions as evaluation data will not always provide valid, reliable data from which to make decisions; however, these may fall under Level 2: Learning of the NWKM, which examines how learners acquire the knowledge, skills, and attitudes from their participation in the SBE, as well as confidence and commitment (Kirkpatrick & Kirkpatrick, 2016).

Reliability and Validity

Evaluation instruments should be reliable and valid for the learner group they are being used for. As an example, if second-semester nursing students are being evaluated on their clinical judgment during a scenario-based activity, then the evaluation instrument should be reliable and valid when used to evaluate clinical judgment of second-semester nursing students. If the instrument has only been tested with second-year medical residents, then it may not be the right choice for nursing students. Reliability means that an instrument will perform the same way each time it is used; it is dependable and trustworthy. For example, stepping on and off the scale three times before a morning shower will give roughly the same result; therefore, the scale is reliable. Validity refers to the accuracy of an assessment instrument when used with certain populations. Does the instrument measure what it is intended to measure? For example, here are three measurement instruments: a ruler, a metal tape measure, and a flexible tape measure. While all three are marked with the same intervals, only one will have valid results when measuring your waist; however, all three would be valid when used to hang a picture on the wall.

TABLE 10.4

Types of Evaluation

Type of Evaluation	How Evaluation Performed	Challenges	Benefits
Self-report measures (e.g., questionnaires, surveys, scales)	Participant reports their own assessment of the construct (e.g., confidence, competence, anxiety, attitudes)	Inaccurate perception Poor self-awareness Unpaired with reality as perceived by the instructor Social desirability bias Response bias Unable to quantify behavior change Missing data can affect analysis	Useful when construct is difficult to visualize or objectively evaluate Anonymous response option Easy data collection method
Behavioral Marker Systems (BMS) (e.g., rating scales, checklists, frequency counts)	Evaluate behaviors and performance objectively by trained observer Data used for evaluation or feedback	Not designed for measuring psychological constructs Resource intensive for training time of observers Cognitive bias Hawthorne effect	Assess technical and nontechnical skills Trained observers Can be used live or with video Standardized/simulated participant can be trained observer
Global Rating Scales	Measures high-level ability to perform a skill, but not specific tasks or components of the skill	Similar to BMS Halo effect Risk artificial inflation of internal consistency of tool	Similar to BMS One rating overall, rather than individual tasks/skills Task-agnostic Can use for variety of skills May be embedded within BMS (Santomauro et al., 2020)
Conversation	Encouraging learners to talk out loud as they participate in scenario Can uncover incorrect thought processes, as can the reflective conversations in debriefing	Lack of sharing due to fear of embarrassment Poor ability to reflect on performance Anxiety	Identify concerns as they occur rather than waiting for debriefing Opportunity to discuss, further reflect in real time Best suited for formative assessment
Haptics, Virtual, and Augmented Reality (VR/AR)	Provide tactile feedback for palpation location, depth of pressure, other types of movements through various tracking devices both internal to the product and external (e.g., glove)	May have prohibitively high cost Low-cost models not durable Low-cost models lack objective evaluation data Moderate sense of haptic feedback (Viglialoro et al., 2021)	Location, depth of pressure documented by machine Found in wearables, VR/AR experiences, game controllers Objective evaluation

One caveat—the instruments must be used as intended. For example, we can move the measuring tape higher on our waist or pull it snugger to alter the results. Educators must be diligent when using evaluation instruments in the way they were intended. Educators need to be able to choose appropriate instruments for evaluation based on reliability and validity and know how to use the instruments appropriately (Santomauro et al., 2020). Further discussion about reliability and validity was included in Chapter 4; educators undertaking high-stakes evaluation must be competent in this area.

High-Stakes Testing

The higher the stakes of the evaluation, the more reliable and valid an instrument must be. Many educators use checklists when signing off on student performance on a task trainer, such as when students are undergoing formative assessment in a weekly skills lab. These checklists may come from textbooks, or websites, or have been created by a nursing educator. If the student does not meet a predetermined number of criteria, then they are assigned further practice. However, at the end of the semester, if the same checklist is used to determine whether a student passes or fails the entire nursing fundamentals program, then the evaluator and the checklist must be held to a higher standard of reliability and validity. When someone's career path depends on the results of the evaluation, three areas must be taken into consideration in addition to the reliability and validity of the evaluation instrument: the design of the experience, the skill of the facilitator, and the competency of the evaluator.

The Healthcare Simulation Standard of Best Practice™ Scenario Design (INACSL Standards Committee, Watts et al., 2021) identified key criteria that must be met if a scenario is to be used for high-stakes testing. Content, or subject matter experts, should help to develop the experience with simulationists with expertise in best practices. A pilot test of the simulation, skills, or SBE must be conducted to be certain the experience accomplishes its purpose. This can be done with students similar to those being tested, such as students from a previous semester. Evaluation methods must be assessed for validity and reliability. The facilitator has responsibility for managing the SBE (INACSL Standards Committee, Persico et al., 2021) and should have initial and ongoing training, as supported by numerous organizations (Alexander et al., 2015; INACSL Standards Committee, Hallmark et al., 2021; Lewis et al., 2017; Society for Simulation in Healthcare [SSH] Accreditation Council, 2022a). It is important that facilitators follow a well-detailed SBE script, in the same manner, for each student participating in a high-stakes exam so there is no variability caused by the facilitator's actions.

Lastly, the evaluator(s) should be formally trained in the use of the instrument used for the high-stakes evaluation so that all evaluators use the instrument in the same way for every student. It is recommended that more than one evaluator is used for each student, either through direct observation or by review of video recordings (INACSL Standards Committee, McMahon et al., 2021). This may require extensive training to establish interrater reliability, depending on the complexity of the instrument. Even a simple dichotomous checklist requires training. For example, consider the student who is being evaluated on communication. Imagine there are three items they are to communicate to a physician, but the student only communicates two of them. If the checklist has a yes (completed) or no (did not complete) option, some evaluators may choose yes because the student

TABLE 10.5

Obtaining a Simulation Evaluation Instrument

Approaches to Obtain a Simulation Evaluation Instrument	Key Points
INACSL Repository of Instruments used in Simulation Research https://www.inacsl.org/repository-of-instruments	Contains a list of instruments sorted according to Jeffries' theory (2016); reliability and validity not noted.
Evaluating Healthcare Simulation website http://sim-eval.org	Free immediate download of various instruments. Well-documented validity and reliability testing. Information on how to use each instrument, as well as establish IRR is available. Some translations are available.
Contact the instrument creator directly	Ask permission to use a copy of the instrument after locating through literature search.
Alter an existing instrument	Consider the impact of reliability and validity if altering an existing instrument. Contact the creator of the instrument prior to adjusting the instrument. For research purposes, seek permission for alterations and re-establish the psychometrics of the instrument.
Create your own instrument.	Time consuming, resource intensive, requires expertise and pilot testing.

completed two of three tasks, while another evaluator will choose no because the task was incomplete. This is even more challenging when using performance rubrics that have a continuum of options (continuous data). Interrater reliability may have to be re-established numerous times during evaluations. It is important that the scenario design, facilitator actions, or evaluator inconsistency is not the cause of learner failure in high-stakes evaluation.

Where to Find Evaluation Instruments

Now that you have followed the steps for determining how to evaluate your students, where do you find a reliable instrument that provides valid data when used with a group like yours? Many articles are published about the psychometric analysis of new instruments, referring to the reliability and validity testing that goes into new instrument development; however, most journal articles do not publish the actual instrument. Table 10.5 provides information about obtaining a simulation evaluation instrument.

ACCREDITATION OF HEALTH CARE SIMULATION PROGRAMS

Further understanding of health care simulation has grown through the use of a common nomenclature (Lioce et al., 2020), standards of best practice for SBE (INACSL Standards

Committee, 2021), use of standardized patients (Lewis et al., 2017), a code of ethics for simulationists (SSH, 2018), a conceptual and operational definition of "excellence" in simulation programs (Palaganas et al., 2015), specialty certification for basic and advanced simulation educators and operations specialists, and accreditation standards for simulation education programs (SSH, 2022a). Quality simulation programs that have established excellent outcomes are able to attain accreditation for their simulation center—a sign of excellence in their work.

ACCREDITATION STANDARDS AND PROCESS

Accreditation is a voluntary process that signifies a dedication to excellence, which affords the accredited program a variety of benefits. Among the benefits to nursing programs are improved education through recognition of best practices, external validation of excellence, and confidence in the program's quality, among others (SSH, 2022a). Standards for accreditation drive the policies and procedures used in a program or organization to ensure quality (Ahmed et al., 2021). During the accreditation process, a delegate of a professional organization gathers and evaluates data about the program to determine how well predetermined quality standards are met (SSH, 2022a).

Over the past 15 years, leaders in simulation have developed standards that define a well-designed simulation program suitable for accreditation. Nursing education simulation program accreditation is offered by SSH, an interprofessional organization that promotes improvements in simulation technology, educational methods, practitioner assessment, and patient safety to provide better patient care and patient outcomes. SSH offers accreditation for health care simulation programs in private industry, hospital, and health professions academic settings. Standards for accreditation are reviewed every five years by a SSH subcommittee to ensure that they follow international trends and emerging evidence.

Simulation programs can earn Core Accreditation, meaning that they meet the fundamental structural and operational standards related to mission and governance, program management, resource management, human resources, program improvement, ethics, and expanding the field of simulation. Programs that apply for Core Accreditation need to apply for accreditation in one additional area: Assessment, Research, or Teaching/Education (SSH, 2022a). Programs that have met requirements for one functional area may add additional areas: Systems Integration and Simulation Fellowship Program.

Assessment

Simulation programs need to demonstrate the ability to develop, implement, and validate summative simulation assessments. To meet this standard for accreditation, evidence of sufficient technology and adequate resources for simulation assessment should be presented. Assessors need to be trained and qualified to use reliable and valid evaluation instruments to gather data about student performance, and there should be sufficient support for the assessment process. Furthermore, evaluation instruments must align with learning objectives. There also needs to be evidence that the assessments reflect the mission and vision of the institution.

Research

To earn accreditation, simulation programs need to provide evidence of data collection, analysis, and dissemination of knowledge related to simulation. There must be organizational and financial commitment to research. Research activities should align with the organization's mission and values. A designated person provides administrative and visionary oversight of simulation research activities. The roles and responsibilities should be clearly described, and a minimum of 20% of the person's time should be dedicated to simulation research. The program needs to show evidence of dissemination of research findings through peer-reviewed publications and presentations. Researchers should be qualified, and collaborative relationships and studies external to the program are expected. Finally, there must be evidence of compliance with ethical requirements for research and sufficient research mentoring.

Teaching/Education

Simulation programs need to demonstrate regular, recurring simulation educational activities with clearly stated objectives (e.g., knowledge, behaviors, and psychomotor skills) to meet the accreditation criteria for Teaching/Education. A clear connection to the mission and vision of the organization and evidence of educational quality improvement should be demonstrated. Evidence must be presented that evidence-based educational activities result from a needs assessment and are designed and implemented in an engaging, effective manner using proper modalities and a level of realism. Qualified educators, who receive ongoing professional development, lead the simulation design, implementation, and evaluation. The simulation program needs to document an orientation process, evaluation, and feedback method for those involved in simulation education. Simulation programs also need to provide evidence of a systematic annual evaluation method for educational activities to ensure learning objectives are met.

TYPES OF ACCREDITATION: PROVISIONAL AND FULL

Provisional Accreditation

Programs with established structures and processes that have not yet documented outcomes can apply for provisional accreditation, which is granted for two years. This allows simulation programs to establish a relationship with the assessor team and receive constructive feedback from these simulation experts to help improve the program, establish a solid foundation, and move it toward full accreditation (SSH, 2022b). Programs seeking provisional accreditation must meet the seven Core Standards but to a lesser extent than required for full accreditation. In addition, the program must demonstrate compliance with the Teaching/Education standards of the chosen area (educational activities, educational activity design, qualified educators, evaluation, and improvement) (Table 10.6).

Full Accreditation

A program is eligible for full SSH accreditation when it has a minimum of two years of experience in the functional area in which accreditation is sought. A program seeking

TABLE 10.6

Full and Provisional Accreditation Overview

CORE STANDARDS
1. Mission & Governance
2. Program Management
3. Resource Management
4. Human Resources
5. Program Improvement
6. Ethics
7. Expanding the Field

Full Accreditation	Provisional
Duration: 5 years	Duration: 2 years
Eligibility: 2 years experience in functional area and evidence of outcomes (SSH, 2022a)	Eligibility: <2 years of simulation, or no evidence of outcomes (SSH, 2022b)
Assessment Standards	Teaching/Education Standards
1. Assessment Activities	1. Educational Activities
2. Assessment Activities Design	2. Educational Activity Design
3. Qualified Assessors	3. Qualified Educators
4. Evaluation and Improvement	4. Evaluation and Improvement
Research Standards	
1. Simulation Research Activities	
2. Simulation Research Activity Design	
3. Qualified Simulation Researchers	
4. Evaluation and Improvement	
5. Simulation Research Collaboration	
6. Compliance	
7. Ethics	
Teaching/Education Standards	
1. Educational Activities	
2. Educational Activity Design	
3. Qualified Educators	
4. Evaluation and Improvement	

Programs that meet the requirements for one functional area can add an additional area:

System Integration
1. Mission & Scope
2. Integration of Activities

Simulation Fellowship Program
1. Program Infrastructure
2. Program Resources
3. Educational Activities
4. Scholarship
5. Program Evaluation & Improvement

full accreditation must demonstrate compliance with the Core Standards and one or more functional areas: Assessment, Research, or Teaching/Education. Programs that have met the requirements for one of these functional areas may elect to add an *additional* area in System Integration and/or Simulation Fellowship Program (SSH, 2022a). The full accreditation period lasts for five years.

LOGISTICS OF ACCREDITATION

The simulation accreditation process is similar to accreditation for nursing programs. The simulation center completes a self-study by using the accreditation standards as a guide, including examples and appendices to summarize data. The accreditation site reviewers study written materials and send clarifying questions prior to the site visit. During the site visit, the reviewers meet with the simulation center team, administration, faculty, and students to determine consistency between the self-study narrative with the policies, procedures, and day-to-day operations of the simulation center.

Timeline

A great deal of time goes into writing a self-study to allow key stakeholders and team members to be involved early in the self-study process. Administrators should be consulted and receive frequent updates. Writing teams must be established, led by those qualified in simulation and possessing good writing and analytical skills. Outlines need to be created and sections assigned to team members to prepare the supporting documents. Working backward from the target submission date, create a timeline that includes review, discussion, and development time (Table 10.7).

Qualified Simulation Educators

Like-minded simulationists are needed to lead the accreditation process. One way to develop simulationists into that role is to offer review courses for best practices in simulation pedagogy. This helps to increase the quality of the SBE and achieve and document the learning outcomes. Simulationists are encouraged to achieve certification in simulation education and operations, which facilitates implementing the Healthcare Simulation Standards of Best Practice (INACSL Standards Committee, 2021) into daily operations. These certifications are offered through the SSH, and they are a cornerstone in building an accredited, high-quality simulation program.

Educators teaching with simulation need to incorporate principles that are unique to simulation pedagogy, such as suspending disbelief among the learners as a simulated scenario and environment are brought "to life," requiring unique knowledge, skills, and abilities. Specific phases of a simulation-based learning experience include designing the scenario, prebriefing, facilitating the simulation, debriefing, and evaluation, each of which requires a deliberately learner-centered perspective.

Preparing Supporting Documents

The SSH self-study tools and Simulation Program Policy and Procedure Model Template (SSH, 2021) aid in cross-matching required policies and procedures to ensure they meet

TABLE 10.7

Typical Timeline to Simulation Accreditation

Activity	Timeline to Full Accreditation Months Prior
Obtain faculty, administration and financial buy-in for pursuing accreditation	>24
Form accreditation writing team and advisory board	24
Review the self-study review tool to assess for current gaps	24
Develop simulation policies and procedures	24
Begin collecting simulation program outcome data	24
Prepare self-study narrative: core standards and at least one functional area	12
Prepare appendices	9
Self-study narrative to dean/administration	4
Obtain consents for images/videos	3
Prepare images/videos of activities	2
Combine narrative, appendices, and images into one electronic document	2
Final edits (editor assistance)	1
Submit self-study (including images/videos/exemplars) to SSH	**Submission Deadline: February 15 and July 15**
Review of self-study and initial responses by SSH	1 month after
SSH clarifying questions/responses	Prior to site visit
SSH site visit	3–5 months after
SSH accreditation board of review	5–8 months after
SSH written feedback and accreditation awarded	1 month after SSH board review
SSH formal recognition at annual conference	Every January
SSH annual reports	Each year

the standards of accreditation and that nothing is overlooked. Important policies related to simulation evaluation need to address confidentiality, psychological safety, and the use of video recordings, among others, prior to any student performance evaluation.

Data collection includes simulation evaluations, equipment inventory, simulation modalities used in the program, and how complaints are handled, among other areas. Data on overall student experiences related to self-confidence and knowledge transfer to clinical practice, student evaluations of simulation effectiveness and attainment of

TABLE 10.8

Example of Simulation Evaluation: Nursing Student Responses on Debriefing Subscale of Simulation Effectiveness Tool—Modified

Item	Strongly Agree n (%)	Somewhat Agree n (%)	Do Not Agree n (%)
1. Debriefing contributed to my learning	167 (86.08)	27 (13.92)	0
2. Debriefing allowed me to communicate my feelings before focusing on the scenario	148 (77.89)	38 (20.00)	4 (2.11)
3. Debriefing was valuable in helping me improve my clinical judgment	161 (84.29)	26 (13.61)	4 (2.09)
4. Debriefing provided opportunities to self-reflect on my performance during simulation	162 (84.38)	25 (13.02)	5 (2.60)
5. Debriefing was a constructive evaluation of the simulation	165 (85.49)	25 (12.95)	3 (1.55)

Source: Leighton, K., Ravert, P., Mudra, V., & Macintosh, C. (2015). Updating the Simulation Effectiveness Tool: Item modifications and reevaluation of psychometric properties. *Nursing Education Perspectives, 36*(5), 317–323. https://doi.org/10.5480/15-1671; Leighton, K, Ravert, P., Mudra, V., & Macintosh, C. (2018). Simulation Effectiveness Tool–Modified. Retrieved from https://sites.google.com/view/evaluatinghealthcaresimulation/set-m.

learning objectives, and evaluations of facilitators and course faculty are all reviewed as part of the continuous quality improvement (CQI) process. An example of an evaluation measuring the effectiveness of debriefing after the simulation is presented in Table 10.8. The data collected for the supporting documents often provide useful information for the administrator to justify the need for additional resources (e.g., manikin, equipment) to be allocated to the simulation center.

Site Visit

The accreditation process includes a site visit to the simulation center. This had been done in person prior to COVID-19 but during the pandemic transitioned to a virtual site visit. When virtual, the self-study submission also includes a video tour of the facility and recorded simulation events (e.g., debriefing). Site visitors may have questions or require clarification of areas of the self-study prior to the visit. In the time between the submission and the site visit, meetings should be held with groups of faculty, staff, students, and administration to review simulation center policies and procedures. The simulation team of nurse educators, technology specialists, and staff can practice answering questions, reviewing policies and procedures, and answering mock reviewer questions. The process of preparing stakeholders for accreditation of the simulation center is similar to preparing for accreditation of the school of nursing as described earlier in Chapter 7.

The day of the visit begins with formal introductions and an agenda review. The reviewers meet with faculty, staff, students, administrators, and other stakeholders, followed by a closed-door deliberation by the SSH accreditation team. At the end of the day, a general session is held where the next steps are explained, including when to expect the final report.

Summary

This chapter provided an overview of the purpose and types of evaluation used in nursing simulation programs, including the numerous constructs that should be evaluated. Several categories of evaluation instruments exist, and the choice of which to use should align with the type of evaluation, learning objectives, and the level of the learner. The facilitator needs to be skilled, incorporate the expertise of subject matter experts, and pilot scenarios to ensure they work properly before using them to evaluate students. Additionally, the facilitator must be trained in both facilitation skills and how to interpret and use the proposed evaluation instrument. Creating a comprehensive simulation program evaluation plan adds to the overall nursing program assessment of learning outcomes.

Accreditation is the next level of achievement for simulation programs that can show excellent outcomes as a result of their evaluation. This achievement brings value to nursing programs by demonstrating the successful use of evidence-based standards leading to quality learning outcomes. Accreditation provides external validation that a program meets benchmarks of best practices in simulation. It is vital to maintain the high standards of providing pedagogically sound SBE. This is possible by continuous and deliberate quality improvement processes, including frequent review of policies, procedures, simulations, evaluation data, and faculty/staff feedback. Providing evaluation data leads to ongoing financial support and the growth of a simulation program.

References

Ahmed, R. A., Wong, A. H., Musits, A. N., Cardell, A., Cassara, M., Wong, N. L., Smith, M. K., Bajaj, K., Meguerdichian, M., & Szyld, D. (2021). Accreditation of simulation fellowships and training programs: More checkboxes or elevating the field? *Simulation in Healthcare.* Advance online publication. https://doi.org/10.1097/SIH.0000000000000593

Alexander, M., Durham, C. F., Hooper, J. I., Jeffries, P. R., Goldman, N., Kardong-Edgren, S., Kesten, K. S., Spector, N., Tagliareni, E., Radtke, B., & Tillman, C. (2015). NCSBN simulation guidelines for prelicensure nursing programs. *Journal of Nursing Regulation, 6*(3), 39–42.

Gaba, D. H. (2004). The future vision of simulation in health care. *Quality and Safety in Health Care, 13*(Suppl 1), i2–i10. https://doi.org/10.1136/qshc.2004.009878

Hayden, J. K., Smiley, R. A., Alexander, M., Kardong-Edgren, S., & Jeffries, P. R. (2014). The NCSBN national simulation study: A longitudinal, randomized, controlled study replacing clinical hours with simulation in prelicensure nursing education. *Journal of Nursing Regulation, 5*(2), C1-S64.

INACSL Standards Committee. (2021). Healthcare Simulation Standards of Best Practice™. *Clinical Simulation in Nursing, 58,* 66. https://doi.org/10.1016/j.ecns.2021.08.018

INACSL Standards Committee, Hallmark, B., Brown, M., Peterson, D., Fey, M., Decker, S., Wells-Beede, E., Britt, T., Hardie, L., Shum, C., Arantes, H. P., Charnetski, M., & Morse, C. (2021). Healthcare Simulation Standards of Best Practice™ Professional Development. *Clinical Simulation in Nursing, 58*, 5–8. https://doi.org/10.1016/j.ecns.2021.08.007

INACSL Standards Committee, McMahon, E., Jimenez, F.A., Lawrence, K. & Victor, J. (2021). Healthcare Simulation Standards of Best Practice™ Evaluation of Learning and Performance. *Clinical Simulation in Nursing, 58*, 54–56. https://doi.org/10.1016/j.ecns.2021.08.016

INACSL Standards Committee, Persico, L., Belle, A., DiGregorio, H., Wilson-Keates, B., & Shelton, C. (2021). Healthcare Simulation Standards of Best Practice™ Facilitation. *Clinical Simulation in Nursing, 58*, 22–26. https://doi.org/10.1016/j.ecns.2021.08.010

INACSL Standards Committee, Watts, P. I., McDermott, D. S., Alinier, G., Charnetski, M., Ludlow, J., Horsley, E., Meakim, C., Nawathe, P. A. (2021). Healthcare Simulation Standards of Best Practice™ Simulation Design. *Clinical Simulation in Nursing, 58*, 14–21. https://doi.org/10.1016/j.ecns.2021.08.009

Jeffries, P. R. (Ed). (2016). *The NLN Jeffries simulation theory*. Wolters Kluwer.

Kirkpatrick, J. D., & Kirkpatrick, W. K. (2016). *Kirkpatrick's four levels of training evaluation*. Association for Talent Development.

Leighton, K. (2017). The evolution of cutting edge technology: Today's simulation typologies. In C. Foisy-Doll & K. Leighton (Eds.), *Simulation champions: Courage, caring and connection* (pp. 70–84). Wolters Kluwer.

Leighton, K., Foisy-Doll, C., Mudra, V., Ravert, P. (2020). Guidance for comprehensive health care simulation program evaluation. *Clinical Simulation in Nursing, 48*(C), 20–28. https://doi.org/10.1016/j.ecns.2020.08.003

Leighton, K., Kardong-Edgren, S., McNelis, A., & Sullo, E. (2022). Learning outcomes attributed to prelicensure clinical education in nursing: A systematic review of qualitative research. *Nurse Educator,* *47*(1), 26–30. https://doi.org/10.1097/NNE.0000000000001097

Leighton, K., Kardong-Edgren, S., McNelis, A. M., Foisy-Doll, C., & Sullo, E. (2021). Traditional clinical outcomes in prelicensure nursing education: An empty systematic review. *Journal of Nursing Education, 60*(3), 136–142. https://doi.org/10.3928/01484834-20210222-03

Leighton, K., Ravert, P., Mudra, V., & Macintosh, C. (2015). Updating the Simulation Effectiveness Tool: Item modifications and reevaluation of psychometric properties. *Nursing Education Perspectives, 36*(5), 317–323. https://doi.org/10.5480/15-1671

Leighton, K, Ravert, P., Mudra, V., & Macintosh, C. (2018). Simulation Effectiveness Tool–Modified. Retrieved from https://sites.google.com/view/evaluatinghealthcaresimulation/set-m

Lewis, K. L., Bohnert, C. A., Gammon, W. L., Hölzer, H., Lyman, L., Smith, C., Thompson, T. M., Wallace, A., Gliva-McConvey, G. (2017). The Association of Standardized Patient Educators (ASPE) Standards of Best Practice (SOBP). *Advances in Simulation, 2,* Article number: 10. https://doi.org/10.1186/s41077-017-0043-4

Lioce, L. (Ed.), Lopreiato, J. (Founding Ed.), Downing, D., Chang, T. P., Robertson, J. M., Anderson, M., Diaz, D. A., Spain. A. E. (Assoc. Eds.), & the Terminology and Concepts Working Group. (2020). *Healthcare simulation dictionary* (2nd ed.). Agency for Healthcare Research and Quality. AHRQ Publication No. 20-0019. doi: https://doi.org/10.23970/simulationv2

Oermann, M. H., & Gaberson, K. B. (2021). *Evaluation and testing in nursing education* (6th ed.). Springer Publishing Company.

Palaganas, J. C., Maxworthy, J. C., Epps, C. A., & Mancini, M. E. (2015). *Defining excellence in simulation programs*. Wolters Kluwer.

Santomauro, C. M., Hill, A., McCurdie, T., & McGlashan, H. L. (2020). Improving the quality of evaluation data in simulation-based healthcare improvement projects. *Simulation in Healthcare, 15*, 341–355. https://doi.org/10.1097/SIH.0000000000000442

Society for Simulation in Healthcare (SSH). (2018). *Healthcare simulationist code of ethics*. https://www.ssih.org/SSH-Resources/Code-of-Ethics

Society for Simulation in Healthcare (SSH). (2021). *SSH Simulation program policy and procedure manual model template*. https://www.ssih.org/Portals/48/Docs/2021/Policy%20Manual%20Template%20v2021.pdf[10].pdf

Society for Simulation in Healthcare (SSH). (2022a). *Full accreditation*. https://www.ssih.org/Credentialing/Accreditation/Full-Accreditation

Society for Simulation in Healthcare (SSH). (2022b). *Provisional accreditation*. https://www.ssih.org/Credentialing/Accreditation/Provisional-Accreditation

Viglialoro, R. M., Condino, S., Turini, G., Carbone, M., Ferrari, V., & Gesi, M. (2021). Augmented reality, mixed reality, and hybrid approach in healthcare simulation: A systematic review. *Applied Science, 11*(5), 2338–2358. https://doi.org/10.3390/app11052338

Evaluation of Education Programs in Practice Settings

Kathy Casey, PhD, RN, NPD-BC

Nursing practice is continuously changing and evolving to keep up with the growing complexity of patient care needs. With the current focus on patient safety and quality outcomes in health care organizations, education programs in practice settings must address professional practice gaps related to clinician knowledge and skill competence, and support role development activities. Effective practice-based education programs have much in common with the development and evaluation of academic nursing education programs. Practice-based education activities and programs are often based on assessed gaps in practice or requests from stakeholders in the organization. To accomplish these education goals, Nursing Professional Development (NPD) practitioners design educational activities to address professional practice gaps for the identified target audience and determine strategies to achieve specific outcomes related to identified deficits or opportunities for improvement in knowledge, skill, or practice (Harper & Maloney, 2022).

This chapter provides an overview of the NPD role, describes the types of practice-based education programs, discusses alignment with the NPD Scope and Standards of Practice competencies to demonstrate program evaluation, and describes the Kirkpatrick model commonly used for program evaluation. Common barriers to evaluating education programs in practice settings are also examined in the chapter.

NURSING PROFESSIONAL DEVELOPMENT PRACTITIONERS

NPD is "a specialized nursing practice that facilitates the professional role development and growth of nurses and other healthcare personnel along the continuum from novice to expert" (Harper & Maloney, 2022, p. 16). NPD practitioners are critical to education program development and implementation and are involved in the evaluation process used to assess the program's quality, effectiveness, and value to the organization. *The Nursing Professional Development: Scope and Standards of Practice* (Harper & Maloney, 2022) outlines the responsibilities and competencies of nurses in professional development roles. These standards provide a framework to document the contributions of NPD in improving professional practice and achieving program goals in healthcare organizations. Clinical Nurse Educators and NPD practitioners are position titles to describe nurses who are responsible for influencing professional role competence and the professional growth of learners in a variety of clinical settings through planning, implementing, and evaluating education programs (Harper & Maloney, 2022). Certification in nursing professional development is a voluntary assessment offered by the American Nurses Credentialing Center (ANCC) to recognize practitioners who have experience in nursing professional development. Certification serves as a measure of knowledge, competence, and excellence in this specialty area of practice.

TYPES OF EDUCATION PROGRAMS IN PRACTICE SETTINGS

Practice-based education programs are important, as they are designed for post-licensed nurses and clinical personnel in health care organizations to ensure staff has the most current, evidence-based knowledge and skills for professional practice. Examples of education programs in practice settings include *Nurse Orientation Programs*, designed to ensure new employees gain information related to the agency mission, regulatory and patient safety policies, acclimate to the culture of the organization, and develop technical expertise on expected skills for the department. These initial training programs vary in length, depending on the type of position and information to be learned.

Preceptor Development Programs are designed to provide education and support for clinical staff to develop the basic knowledge, skills, and abilities necessary to function in the preceptor role. These programs offer opportunities for professional growth in learning the skills and competencies needed to guide the new employee to gain both the skill and confidence to function independently in today's demanding work environment (Cotter & Dienemann, 2016).

Charge Nurse Leadership Training Programs have been developed in recent years. This training is desirable as charge nurses are the designated leaders when nurse managers are not available. Since charge nurses provide leadership for staff and support for patients and visitors on their unit or department, the training includes how charge nurses use various measurements (e.g., quality metrics, staff satisfaction) to evaluate unit effectiveness of the units, from quality measures to staff satisfaction (Bateman & King, 2020).

Implementation of a *Clinical Ladder Program* is a strategy used by many health care institutions to quantify and promote the professional development of bedside nurses (Meucci, Moore, & McGrath, 2019). These programs promote financial incentives, raise job satisfaction, aid in recruitment and retention of staff, and recognize nurses for advanced performance (Hespenheide, Cottingham, & Mueller, 2011).

To retain graduate nurses, health care institutions are following the National Academy of Medicine's (2011) recommendation to implement *Nurse Residency Programs* to facilitate graduate nurse transition to practice and reduce nurse turnover. These programs have been developed and embraced as an innovative intervention to provide support for newly graduated nurses as they transition into practice, increase clinical competency in the professional role, improve confidence and job satisfaction, and improve graduate nurse retention (Goode et al., 2013; Goode et al., 2016).

Accreditation of nurse residency programs is a relatively new process and is a voluntary activity. Accreditation of nurse residency programs began with the Commission on Collegiate Nursing Education (CCNE) in 2008. The CCNE standards require an academic-practice partnership that strengthens the understanding of how new nurses are prepared academically and how they are applying that knowledge to practice (CCNE, 2021). The CCNE standards were amended in 2015. In 2014, the ANCC Practice Transition Accreditation Program standards were developed for residency and fellowship programs. Common elements among transition to practice program standards include the structure of the program (hospital or organization demographics, number of nurse residents, and human, physical, and financial resources); the process (curriculum, preceptor-based practice, and competency development); and the outcomes (retention, confidence, satisfaction, and professional development) (Church et al., 2019).

Careful attention to accreditation standards and requirements are important details to be included in an evaluation of nurse residency programs. Accreditation criteria have been established to assist in reducing nurse residency program variability and help ensure best practices in the development and support of newly licensed graduate nurses. Accreditation standards require current, reliable, and valid evaluation methods to demonstrate program quality and measure outcomes (ANCC, 2015). The appropriate selection of measurement instruments and the extent to which their reliability and validity are demonstrated have a profound influence on the strength of the findings. The measurement tool most frequently used in published studies to measure graduate nurses self-reported perceptions of the transition to practice experience is the Casey-Fink Graduate Nurse Experience Survey (Casey et al., 2004; Stephenson & Cosme, 2018). Using a valid and reliable measurement tool allows health care organizations to compare their results with other organizations using the same population of interest.

EDUCATION PROGRAM EVALUATION ALIGNMENT WITH NPD SCOPE AND STANDARDS

Program evaluation is an integral part of the education design process to determine whether the professional practice gap and learner outcomes were met and if there has been an effect on practice (Schumacher et al., 2018). A systematic process for evaluating practice-based education programs is needed to ensure the effectiveness of delivery, discover if the outcomes were achieved, and establish the overall effect on the learners and the organization.

Practice-based education programs, similar to academic education programs, need an in-depth process to assess if the interventions in these programs are having the desired effect. As health care organizations shift to an outcomes-based approach to care, it is important that NPD practitioners set clear goals and outcomes for education programs to assist in measuring program success for their stakeholders. Establishing a program evaluation plan, which includes a data collection plan, can be helpful in making program revisions and improving program outcomes. Standard 6 of the *Nursing Professional Development: Scope and Standard of Practice* (Harper & Maloney, 2022) addresses program evaluation, which includes the expectation that NPD practitioners formulate

BOX 11.1

Standard 6. Nursing Professional Development: Scope and Standards of Practice: Competencies of the NPD Practitioner

1. Conducts systematic and ongoing evaluation of the expected outcomes of the prescribed plan.
2. Uses appropriate methods and instruments to measure outcomes.
3. Creates opportunities for feedback on and evaluation of the effectiveness of the plan, including strategies used and the influences of the interprofessional practice and learning environments.
4. Involves learners and stakeholders in the evaluation process.
5. Analyzes the evaluation data.
6. Documents the outcomes of NPD initiatives.
7. Revises NPD initiatives based on evaluation data.
8. Disseminates the evaluation results to relevant stakeholders.
9. Identifies opportunities to overcome barriers to sustain expected outcomes.
10. Creates processes to identify and involve stakeholders in the evaluation process.
11. Formulates a systematic and effective ongoing evaluation plan aimed at measuring processes and outcomes that are relevant to NPD initiatives, learners, and stakeholders.
12. Uses valid, reliable, and relevant methods and instruments to measure behavior change and impact.
13. Synthesizes evaluation data to guide decision-making about ongoing and future NPD initiatives.
14. Synthesizes evaluation data to determine the plan's impact on healthcare consumer(s)/ partner(s) and population health, as appropriate.
15. Analyzes NPD initiatives' value based on achieved outcomes.
16. Leads dissemination of evaluation data to key stakeholders.
17. Uses results of evaluation to recommend and conduct research, process, policy, procedure, or protocol revisions when warranted.

an evaluation plan, use reliable and valid instruments to measure processes and outcomes, involve learner and stakeholders in the evaluation process, synthesize evaluation data to guide decision-making about educational programming, revise learning activities based on evaluation data, disseminate evaluation results of learning activities, and demonstrate program value based on achieved outcomes. These competencies frame the expected behaviors for NPD practitioners to demonstrate when evaluating educational activities and programs in the practice setting. Expected competencies of the NPD practitioner are delineated in Box 11.1.

Formulating an evaluation plan begins by reviewing the defined program goals and outcomes. Outcome measurement enables NPD practitioners to evaluate evidence to determine whether educational activities closed the gaps in nurses' knowledge, skill, and/or practice (Pepsnik, 2017). Examples of program outcomes include program completion rates, program satisfaction scores, turnover or retention rates.

To measure the outcomes of educational activities and programs, evaluation tools must be reliable, valid, and meaningful (Pepsnik, 2017). Furthermore, NPD practitioners should use multiple instruments that measure a variety of outcomes and attempt to measure outcomes at all four levels of the Kirkpatrick model (Kirkpatrick & Kirkpatrick, 2016; Stephenson & Cosme, 2018). Evaluation tools can be used formatively throughout the educational activity and in the summative evaluation at the culmination of the education program (Cardwell, 2020). Formative evaluations are used during classroom or simulation instruction to assess delivery of content, expertise of the faculty, teaching methods, and whether participants can apply what they learned in practice. Collecting formative assessment data and feedback is used to appraise the effectiveness of learning strategies, the extent to which learners are grasping the knowledge presented, and the need for additional clarification of the material. Summative evaluations are used to appraise teaching effectiveness, determine the effectiveness of instructional strategies and learning activities, and guide revisions to the education program. These evaluations are intended to assess the overall satisfaction or merit of the program.

Engagement of program stakeholders and learners is critical to have a highly successful education program. Including learners, leaders, and stakeholders is needed to set clear goals based on factors such as organizational values, program purpose, and the ability to demonstrate intrinsic or financial value (Taylor & Hall, 2017). These multiple stakeholders have a vested interest in ensuring health care professionals remain competent.

NPD practitioners rely on collected evidence to determine whether an education activity has resulted in closure or reduction in knowledge, skill, or practice gaps. Changes to the program curriculum and learning activities are made based on the data analysis. It is important to document the programmatic changes made and to share the outcomes with leadership and stakeholder teams. Establishing a timeline for data collection (e.g., baseline, midway, and post-program) is important to demonstrate improvement in program outcomes. Frequent feedback and reporting of program outcome data to the organization's nursing leadership are essential.

EDUCATION PROGRAM EVALUATION MODEL

The Kirkpatrick Model of Evaluation, New World Kirkpatrick Model introduced in Chapter 10, and other adaptations of the Kirkpatrick Model are commonly used to evaluate the effectiveness of training programs and education activities (Kirkpatrick & Kirkpatrick, 2006; Kirkpatrick & Kirkpatrick, 2016). The Kirkpatrick Model provides a useful roadmap that integrates evaluation into the initial planning process (DeSilets, 2018). This model includes four levels for evaluation:

1. Reaction, measures reactions of participants to the program or activity (usually information provided at the end).
2. Learning, measures the knowledge or skill that has been acquired during the learning activity.
3. Behavior, provides helpful information on how or whether participants have been able to use or apply what they have learned in practice.
4. Results, collects data on long-term outcomes, and the impact of the learning on the organization.

Level 1 Reaction	• Measures the learner's reaction or satisfaction with the education or training • Evaluation methods - participant surveys, formative and summative evaluations, focus groups, and faculty interviews
Level 2 Learning	• Measures the extent of learning • Evaluation methods - tests, portfolio, journaling, role-play, return demonstration, case study, and simulation
Level 3 Behavior	• Measures the learner's behavior change after the education or training • Evaluation methods - observation of performance, self-report, medical record audit, and competency assessment tools
Level 4 Results	• Measures tangible long-term outcomes that can be directly related to the education or training • Evaluation methods - quality metrics, risk management metrics, employee turnover or retention metrics, length of orientation, program completion rates, reduction in errors, and financial impact

FIGURE 11.1 Kirkpatrick's four levels of training evaluation. *Source:* Kirkpatrick, D. L. (2006). Seven keys to unlock the four levels of evaluation. *Performance Improvement, 45*(7), 5–8; Association for Nursing Professional Development (2017). Nursing Professional Development Certification Preparation Course. ANPD.

A synthesis of the model and methods to evaluate at each level are articulated in a flow diagram to demonstrate how program evaluation can be operationalized. This diagram is shown in Figure 11.1. Liu et al. (2019) used the Kirkpatrick Model to evaluate the effectiveness of a redesigned preceptor education program using three different tools to measure reaction, learning, and behaviors. Using the Kirkpatrick model for planning the evaluation begins with level 4, then moves back to level 3, before going to level 2, and then level 1 (DeSilets, 2018).

BARRIERS TO EDUCATION PROGRAM EVALUATION IN PRACTICE SETTINGS

As with many programs, there are barriers to implementing data collection and analysis for outcome measures in program evaluation (Taylor & Hall, 2017). These include a lack of organizational readiness for change, the organization's culture may not support newly learned behaviors, and the NPD practitioner may lack skills in data analysis. In addition, even though NPD practitioners know the importance that outcomes have in proving value and effectiveness, some find it not worth the cost to do the work (Taylor & Hall, 2017). A proactive approach to facilitating effective educational activities includes anticipating organizational barriers, involving stakeholders in program planning, and remaining flexible and nimble when adapting to the demands of a rapidly changing health care environment.

Summary

Establishing a comprehensive program evaluation plan for education programs in the practice setting is critical to demonstrate the program's impact on learners and their practice, improve program effectiveness, and demonstrate the program's value to the health care organization. Establishing outcome measures that are clearly defined and agreed on by the NPD practitioners and organizational stakeholders is essential to measuring the effectiveness and efficacy of the program process improvement activities.

References

American Nurses Credentialing Center. (2015). 2015 ANCC primary accreditation provider application manual (Riv. 1). Retrieved June 15, 2022 from https://www.nursingworld. org/_4b0217/globalassets/docs/ancc/manuals/ancc-2530-ncpd-applicant-journey-toolkit-final-v-1.0-9.27.21.pdf Author.

Association for Nursing Professional Development. (2017). Nursing Professional Development Certification Preparation Course. Retrieved June 15, 2022 from https://www.anpd.org/page/certification-preparation Author.

Bateman, J. M., & King, S. (2020). Charge nurse leadership training comparison: Effective and timely delivery. *Pediatric Nursing*, 46(4), 189–195.

Cardwell, L. J. (2020). Engaging learners in the evaluation process. *Journal of Continuing Education in Nursing*, 51(4), 149–150. doi:10.3928/00220124-20200317-02

Casey, K., Fink, R., Krugman, M., & Propst, J. (2004). The graduate nurse experience. *Journal of Nursing Administration*, 34(6), 303–311. doi: 10.1097/00005110-20040600000010

Church, C. D., Cosme, S., & O'Brien, M. (2019). Accreditation of transition to practice programs. *Journal for Nurses in Professional Development*, 35(4), 180–184. doi: 10.1097/NND.0000000000000555

Commission on Collegiate Nursing Education. (2021). Standards for accreditation of entry to practice nurse residency programs. https://www.aacnnursing.org/Portals/42/CCNE/PDF/Procedures-Residency.pdf

Cotter, E., & Dienemann, J. (2016). Professional development of preceptors improves nurse outcomes. *Journal for Nurses in Professional Development*, 32(4), 192–197. doi: 10.1097/NND.0000000000000266

DeSilets, L. D. (2018). An update on Kirkpatrick's model of evaluation: Part two. *Journal of Continuing Education in Nursing*, 49(7), 292–293. doi: 10.3928/00220124-20180613-02

Goode, C. J., Lynn, M. R., McElroy, D., Bednash. G. D., & Murray, B. (2013). Lessons learned from 10 years of research on a post-baccalaureate nurse residency program. *Journal of Nursing Administration*, 43(2), 71–77. doi.org/10.1097/nna.0b013e31827f205c

Goode, C. J., Ponte, P. R., & Havens, D. S. (2016). Residency for transition into practice. *Journal of Nursing Administration*, 46(2), 82–86. doi:10.1097/NNA.0000000000000300

Harper, M. G., & Maloney, P. (Eds.). (2022). *Nursing professional development: Scope and standards of practice* (4th ed.). Association for Nursing Professional Development.

Hespenheide, M., Cottingham, T., & Mueller, G. (2011). Portfolio use as a tool to demonstrate professional development in advanced nursing practice. *Clinical Nurse Specialist*, 25(6), 312–320. doi:10.1097/NUR.0b013e318233ea90

Kirkpatrick, D. L. (2006). Seven keys to unlock the four levels of evaluation. *Performance Improvement*, 45(7), 5–8.

Kirkpatrick, D. L., & Kirkpatrick, J. D. (2006). *Evaluating training programs: The four levels* (3rd ed.). Berrett-Koehler.

Kirkpatrick, J. D., & Kirkpatrick, W. K. (2016). *Kirkpatrick's four levels of training evaluation.* Association for Talent Development.

Liu, L., Fillipucci, D., & Mahajan, S. M. (2019). Quantitative analyses of the effectiveness of a newly designed preceptor workshop. *Journal for Nurses in Professional Development, 35*(3), 144–151. DOI: 10.1097/NND.0000000000000528

Meucci, J., Moore, A., & McGrath, J. M. (2019). Testing evidence-based strategies for clinical ladder program refinement. *Journal of Nursing Administration, 49*(11), 561–568. doi: 10.1097/NNA.0000000000000812

National Academy of Medicine. (2011). *The future of nursing: Leading change, advancing health.* National Academies Press.

Pepsnik, D. (2017). Measuring outcomes at the activity level. In P. S. Dickerson (Ed.), *Core curriculum for nursing professional development* (5th ed., pp. 198–206). Association for Nursing Professional Development.

Schumacher, C., Shinners, L., & Graebe, J. (2018). Evaluating the effectiveness of educational activities: Part one. *Journal of Continuing Education in Nursing, 49*(6), 245–247. doi: 103928100220124-240180517-02

Stephenson, J. K., & Cosme, S. (2018). Instruments to evaluate nurse residency programs: A review of the literature. *Journal for Nurses in Professional Development, 34*(3), 123–132. doi: 10.1097/NND.0000000000000444

Taylor, S., & Hall, S. (2017). Measuring success: Goals and outcomes for educational programs. *Journal of Continuing Education in Nursing, 48*(12), 537–538. doi:10.3928/00220124-20171115-02

Examples of Completed Evaluation Plans

TABLE A.1

Completed Evaluation Plan for Faculty and Student Participation in Program Governance

Evaluation Plan Criterion:

ACEN, 1.2: The governing organization and nursing education unit ensure representation of the nurse administrator and nursing faculty in governance activities; opportunities exist for student representation in governance activities.

CCNE, I-E: Faculty and students participate in program governance.

CNEA, II-B: The organizational structure of the parent institution and the nursing program provide opportunities for faculty and students to demonstrate involvement in institutional and program governance, enabling achievement of expected program outcomes.

Persons Responsible	Expected Level of Achievement	Method for Assessment	Timeframe for Evaluation	Actions Taken
Committee chairs (for reporting participation). Department chairs (for ensuring faculty representation). Program directors (for ensuring student representation).	80% of full-time faculty will be members of standing committees in nursing program. 50% of full-time faculty will be members of standing committees at the parent institution level. At least two standing committees in the nursing program will have students as members and will document student participation.	Committee chair reports and minutes showing participation Committee rosters	At end of academic year (May).	Department chairs contacted to increase faculty participation in university committees. Committee chairs of the three committees that include students asked to brainstorm ways to increase student participation in committee business.

Aggregate results for this year: Partially met.

Per School committee roster, 3 of 8 standing committees (Curriculum, Evaluation, Student affairs) list students as members. Minutes show that students attended and participated in 25% of Evaluation committee meetings, 10% of Curriculum committee meetings, and 50% of Student affairs committee meetings.

Per School committee roster, 45 of 50 full-time faculty members are members of standing committees.

Per University committee roster, 20 of 50 full-time nursing faculty members are members of university committees.

TABLE A.2

Completed Evaluation Plan for Faculty Expertise Criterion

Evaluation Plan Criterion:

ACEN, 2.6: Faculty (full- and part-time) maintain expertise in their areas of responsibility, and their performance reflects scholarship and evidence-based teaching and clinical practices.

CCNE, II-E: Faculty are: sufficient in number to accomplish the mission, goals, and expected program outcomes; academically prepared for the areas in which they teach; and experientially prepared for the areas in which they teach.

CNEA, III-D: Faculty demonstrate individual and collective achievement of the program's expected faculty outcomes.

Persons Responsible	Expected Level of Achievement	Method for Assessment	Timeframe for Evaluation	Actions Taken
Department Chairs	100% of full- and part-time faculty will be academically and experientially qualified for the areas in which they teach upon hire.	Transcripts and CVs at time of hire.	At end of academic year (May).	Continue to monitor.
Faculty	100% of full- and part-time faculty will be evaluated annually based upon performance criteria appropriate for their rank and track.	Faculty members' individual annual reports.		
	50% of full-time faculty will demonstrate a scholarship activity during the academic year.	Department chair aggregates annual reports.		
	75% of full- and part-time faculty will demonstrate evidence-based teaching practices during the academic year.	Faculty evaluations conducted by department chairs.		
	90% of full- and part-time faculty teaching clinical courses will document clinical practice experience during the past two years.			

Aggregate results for this year: Met.

Four new full-time and one new part-time faculty members hired in AY 20–21, all met academic and experiential requirements for position.

Department chairs report that all full- and part-time faculty submitted annual reports and received a performance evaluation during AY 20–21.

30 of 50 (60%) full-time faculty members documented a scholarship activity appropriate to their track and rank on their 2020–2021 annual report.

45 of 50 (90%) and 10 of 12 (83%) part-time faculty documented evidence-based teaching on their 2020–2021 annual report.

100% of full- and part-time faculty teaching clinical courses during AY 20–21 document clinical practice experience from 2019–2021.

TABLE A.3

Completed Evaluation Plan for Assessment of Student Complaints

Evaluation Plan Criterion:

ACEN, 3.7: Records reflect that program complaints and grievances receive due process and include evidence of resolution.

CCNE, I-G: The program defines and reviews formal complaints according to established policies.

CNEA, IV-D: Faculty and staff process the formal program complaints of students using policies and procedures that are clearly delineated.

Persons Responsible	Expected Level of Achievement	Method for Assessment	Timeframe for Evaluation	Actions Taken
Program directors	Student complaint policy and procedure listed in all student handbooks and on nursing program website.	Student handbooks	At end of academic year (May).	Continue to monitor.
Associate dean for student affairs	Program directors report student complaints and resolution in annual reports to associate dean for student affairs.	Program director annual reports of student complaints and resolution.		
Dean	Dean of nursing program submits formal complaint log to university annually.	Dean report of formal complaint log to university.		

Aggregate results for this year: Met.

100% of student handbooks contain the formal complaint policy and procedure. Nursing website contains link to formal complaint policy and procedure.

Per program director report, 3 formal complaints were submitted during AY 20–21 from the BSN program. All complaints resolved within the nursing program chain of command. No formal complaints received from other nursing programs.

Dean submitted formal complaint log to university on 5/31/21.

TABLE A.4

Completed Evaluation Plan for Assessment of Curriculum by Faculty

Evaluation Plan Criterion:

ACEN, 4.3: The curriculum is developed by the faculty and regularly reviewed to ensure integrity, rigor, and currency.

CCNE, III-J: The curriculum and teaching-learning practices are evaluated at regularly scheduled intervals and evaluation data are used to foster ongoing improvement.

CNEA, V-J: There is systematic and ongoing review and evidence-based revision of the curriculum and teaching, learning, and evaluation strategies by faculty within a culture of continuous quality improvement to foster achievement of the program's expected student outcomes.

Persons Responsible	Expected Level of Achievement	Method for Assessment	Timeframe for Evaluation	Actions Taken
Program faculty and directors	Program faculty and directors will discuss the curriculum annually during at least one faculty meeting.	Program faculty meeting minutes. Curriculum committee plan for systematic curriculum review.	At end of academic year (May)	Continue to monitor BSN program. Send reminder to MSN program director to schedule discussion of curriculum during at least one faculty meeting in AY 21–22.
Curriculum committee	Curriculum committee will review each course/program curriculum every two years using a checklist and provide feedback to faculty/program directors.	Curriculum committee minutes. Curriculum committee chair annual report.		

Aggregate results for this year: Partially met.

Review of BSN program faculty meeting minutes show that the curriculum courses and plan were discussed on 10/3/20 and 4/5/21.

Review of MSN program faculty meeting minutes show course reports, but no formal discussion of curriculum as a whole.

Curriculum committee reviewed the MSN program during AY 20–21 per their systematic curriculum review plan. Per curriculum committee minutes and chair annual report, the MSN courses were found to be current and to contain appropriate teaching-learning strategies and evaluation methods. A report was sent to the MSN program director of the curriculum committee review to be shared with the faculty.

TABLE A.5

Completed Evaluation Plan for Assessment of Physical Resources

Evaluation Plan Criterion:

ACEN, 5.2: Physical resources are sufficient to ensure the achievement of the end-of-program student learning outcomes and program outcomes, and meet the needs of the faculty, staff, and students.

CCNE, II-B: Physical resources and clinical sites enable the program to fulfill its mission, goals, and expected outcomes. Adequacy of physical resources and clinical sites are reviewed periodically and resources are modified as needed.

CNEA, II-G: Nursing program resources are periodically reviewed and allocated as needed to sustain an environment of continuous quality improvement that enables the program to meet expected program outcomes and expected student learning outcomes.

Persons Responsible	Expected Level of Achievement	Method for Assessment	Timeframe for Evaluation	Actions Taken
Associate dean for operations Program directors Students	Associate dean for operations will report that the physical resources are adequate for delivery of courses and other nursing program needs. Program directors will report that physical resources are adequate for all program activities. 85% of students will state they are satisfied or highly satisfied with the physical resources of the nursing program, on their end-of-program surveys.	Associate dean for operations annual report. Program directors annual report. End-of-program surveys given to graduating students in all programs.	At end of academic year (May).	Continue to monitor program.

Aggregate results for this year: Met.

Associate dean for operations annual report states that all classrooms and conference rooms were adequate for courses and meetings scheduled in the nursing building during AY 20–21.

Program directors state that faculty reported that all rooms and equipment were adequate to deliver courses in the nursing building during AY 20–21.

90% of graduating students (75% response rate) stated they were satisfied or highly satisfied on the end-of-program surveys.

TABLE A.6

Completed Evaluation Plan for Graduate Employment Criterion

Evaluation Plan Criterion:

ACEN, 6.4: The program demonstrates evidence of graduates' achievement in job placement.

CCNE, IV-E: Employment rates demonstrate program effectiveness.

CNEA, I-E: The program achieves expected program outcomes related to graduate employment rates in the area of nursing program preparation.

Persons Responsible	Expected Level of Achievement	Method for Assessment	Timeframe for Evaluation	Actions Taken
Associate dean for student affairs.	80% of graduates will be employed in a nursing position in the area of preparation by 9 months after graduation.	Associate dean for student affairs annual report. Responses from graduate employment surveys.	9 months after May graduation (February).	Continue to monitor employment rates. Ask program directors to remind students during the last course of the importance of completing employment surveys.

Aggregate results for this year: Met.

Pre-licensure BSN program: 90% employed in positions requiring RN licensure (80% response rate for survey).

RN-BSN program: 97% employed in positions requiring RN licensure (40% response rate for survey).

MSN program: 85% employed in nursing position requiring advanced degree (55% response rate for survey).

167